I0014101

JOURNAL OF GREEN ENGINEERING

Aims and Scopes
Journal of Green Engineering will publish original, high quality, peer-reviewed research papers and review articles dealing with environmentally safe engineering including their systems. Paper submission is solicited on:

- Theoretical and numerical modeling of environmentally safe electrical engineering devices and systems.
- Simulation of performance of innovative energy supply systems including renewable energy systems, as well as energy harvesting systems.
- Modeling and optimization of human environmentally conscientiousness environment (especially related to electromagnetics and acoustics).
- Modeling and optimization of applications of engineering sciences and technology to medicine and biology.
- Advances in modeling including optimization, product modeling, fault detection and diagnostics, inverse models.
- Advances in software and systems interoperability, validation and calibration techniques. Simulation tools for sustainable environment (especially electromagnetic, and acoustic).
- Experiences on teaching environmentally safe engineering (including applications of engineering sciences and technology to medicine and biology).

All these topics may be addressed from a global scale to a microscopic scale, and for different phases during the life cycle.

JOURNAL OF GREEN ENGINEERING

Volume 1   No. 4   August 2011

Editorial Foreword   v–vi

FERNANDO J. VELEZ, MARIA DEL CAMINO NOGUERA,
OLIVER HOLLAND and A. HAMID AGHVAMI / Fixed
WiMAX Profit Maximisation with Energy Saving through
Relay Sleep Modes and Cell Zooming   355–381

KOSTAS TSAGKARIS, GEORGE ATHANASIOU, MARIOS
LOGOTHETIS, YIOULI KRITIKOU, DIMITRIOS KAR-
VOUNAS and PANAGIOTIS DEMESTICHAS / Introducing
Energy Awareness in the Cognitive Management of Future
Networks   383–412

S. MANDZUKA, Z. KLJAIĆ and P. ŠKORPUT / The Use of Mo-
bile Communication in Traffic Incident Management Process   413–429

ENRICO   PAOLINI,   ANDREA   GIORGETTI,   SIMONE
MINARDI and MARCO CHIANI / A Heterogenous Network
for Energy Metering and Control   431–445

PAVEL SOMOVAT and VINOD NAMBOODIRI / Energy Consumption of Personal Computing Including Portable Communication Devices   447–475

IRENA OROVIĆ, NIKOLA ŽARIĆ, SRDJAN STANKOVIĆ,
IGOR RADUSINOVIĆ and ZORAN VELJOVIĆ / Analysis of
Power Consumption in OFDM Systems   477–489

Author Index   491–492

Keywords Index   493–494

Editorial Foreword

Dina Simunic[1] and Ramjee Prasad[2]

[1]Faculty of Electrical Engineering and Computing, University of Zagreb, Croatia
[2]CTIF, Aalborg University, Denmark

Dear Reader,

We are very happy to announce the fourth issue of the *Journal of Green Engineering* This issue presents six papers, which all cover very interesting and timely topics in the field of green engineering. The first paper by F.J. Velez, M. del Camino Noguera, O. Holland and A. Hamid Aghvami, entitled "Fixed WiMAX Profit Maximisation with Energy Saving through Relay Sleep Modes and Cell Zooming", shows that the application of cell zooming in conjunction with relays going into sleep mode at times of low load achieves a notable power saving, corresponding to a 10% saving in operation and maintenance cost on average. The second paper by K. Tsagkaris, G. Athanasiou, M. Logothetis, Y. Kritikou, D. Karvounas and P. Demestichas, entitled "Introducing Energy Awareness in the Cognitive Management of Future Networks", describes technologies as important elements in the design of energy-aware future networks. The paper by S. Mandžuka, Z. Kljaić and P. Škorput, "The Use of Mobile Communication in Traffic Incident Management Process", gives a description of incident management system technology, known as the Cell Broadcasting, used in intelligent transport systems. E. Paolini, A. Giorgetti, S. Minardi and M. Chiani in the paper "A Heterogeneous Network for Energy Metering and Control" reveal how proposed methodologies permit the measurement of the consumption of gas, energy, water, etc., in an urban scenario with a large number of nodes, and to remotely control the lighting system for efficient energy usage, together with the description of the successfully implemented testbed. P. Somavat and V. Namboodiri in "Energy Consumption of Personal Computing Including Portable Communication Devices" quantify the impact of energy consumed by the computing sector on the environment, and the cost of electricity for an average residential consumer, together with the provided recommendations for the computer networking community for sustainable portable/mobile computing. The final paper in this issue by I. Orović, N. Žarić, S. Stanković, I. Radusinović and Z. Veljović on "Analysis of Power Consumption in OFDM Systems" provides a comparative study that can be used for an optimal system selection with predefined power consumption requirements.

In addition, we are pleased to inform you that the *Journal of Green Engineering* was the official journal and media sponsor of the *34th International Convention on Information and Communication Technology, Electronics and Microelectronics – MIPRO 2011*, which was held in Opatija, Croatia, 23–27 May 2011, with approximately 1200 participants from all over the world.

Thank you all very much for your kind support of the "Green Engineering" idea and for your active cooperation!

Respectfully,
with our best wishes,

Dina and Ramjee

Fixed WiMAX Profit Maximisation with Energy Saving through Relay Sleep Modes and Cell Zooming

Fernando J. Velez,[1] Maria del Camino Noguera,[1] Oliver Holland[2] and A. Hamid Aghvami[2]

[1]*Instituto de Telecomunicações, DEM, Faculdade de Engenharia, Universidade da Beira Interior, 6201-001 Covilhã, Portugal;*
e-mail: fjv@ubi.pt, maria.noguera02@alu.umh.es;
[2]*Centre for Telecommunications Research, King's College London, Strand, London WC2R 2LS, United Kingdom;*
e-mail: oliver.holland@kcl.ac.uk, hamid.aghvami@kcl.ac.uk

Received: 5 May 2011; Accepted: 6 June 2011

Abstract

In Fixed WiMAX, the cost/revenue optimisation function for radio and network planning incorporates the cost of building and maintaining the infrastructure and the impact of the available resources on revenues. Supported throughput typically decreases with larger cells due to the implied greater average distance of users from the base station, although the use of subchannelisation can keep throughput steady with a larger cell radius. The use of sectored base stations facilitates selection of higher order modulation and coding schemes in the cell and can improve throughput; however, sectored equipment is more expensive. Fortuitously, using Relay Stations (RSs) can reduce the deployment cost of such systems. In such a context, if RSs are put into sleep mode during the night and at weekends when they are not necessary, important energy savings can be achieved. With relays, only the consideration of tri-sectored Base Station (BS) antennas with $K = 3$ (at the cost of extra channels, where nine channels corresponds to a bandwidth of 31.5 MHz) obtains values of system throughput comparable to those without

Journal of Green Engineering, 355–381.

using relays. This is due to the more favourable frame format that is employed under the use of tri-sectored BS antennas.

This paper shows that the application of cell zooming in conjunction with relays going into sleep mode at times of low load achieves a notable power saving, corresponding to 10% saving in operation and maintenance cost on average. Moreover, as it is assumed that the DL sub-frame format cannot be changed to a more favourable one, economic performance is better when RSs are deployed. It is however important to highlight that in the absence of RSs, economic performance is still reasonable (for tri-sectored and omnidirectional BSs, 700–800% and 400–450% profit, respectively), compared with the case where RSs are deployed (~1000 and ~900% profit, respectively).

Keywords: broadband communication, WiMAX, planning, economics, relays, green communications, cell zooming.

1 Introduction

To complement landline services, the demand for multimedia (MM) service delivery through broadband wireless access (BWA) is gaining momentum from both subscribers and service providers. This next step in wireless communications provides ubiquitous Internet and large bandwidth. In order to create conditions for an efficient technology, addressing interoperability and competition in this promising market, a standardisation effort has been led by the Institute of Electrical and Electronic Engineers (IEEE). The first released standard was the IEEE 802.16, which addresses a wide range of frequencies, and defines the main principles for the series of the IEEE 802.16 fixed wireless and mobile standards published afterwards [1, 2]. The advanced air interface of IEEE 802.16m will enable multi-hop relay architectures, roaming and seamless connectivity across IMT-advanced and IMT-2000 systems through the use of appropriate interworking functions.

Worldwide interoperability for Microwave Access (WiMAX) is the commercial name for IEEE 802.16. WiMAX is a BWA technology capable of delivering voice, video, data and MM over the microwave RF spectrum to stationary or moving users.

In the optimisation of cellular planning for fixed WiMAX, the use of Relay Stations (RSs) makes unnecessary a wire-line backhaul, improving significantly coverage whilst achieving competitive values for the system capacity (although slightly lower throughput is achieved). RSs have much lower hardware complexity and using them may significantly reduce the deployment cost of the system as well as its energy consumption: these reasons justify the need for optimisation of fixed WiMAX networks with relays. The motivation to carry out this research work was to optimize the method to obtaining curves for carrier-to-noise-plus-interference, CNIR, vs. distance and the maximum supported throughput by considering different modulation and coding schemes (MCSs) for all possible frequency reuse patterns, e.g., $K = 1$, 3 and 7. A modelling approach is followed by the computation of CNIR and supported throughput. By weighting the physical throughput achieved in each concentric cell coverage ring by the size of the ring, the contribution from each transmission mode (or MCS) is included in an implicit function formulation to obtain the average supported throughput. For consecutive MCSs, the step distances are determined by looking at the correspondence between the minimum feasible values of the CNIR curves (for a given MCS), and the supported throughput, through an inversion procedure.

A comparison of the different values of achieved throughput is performed between the RSs, Base Stations (BSs) and Subscriber Stations (SSs). In the presence of relays, the frames need to guarantee resources for BS-to-SS communications but also for BS-to-RS and RS-to-SS communications. As there usually is less traffic load in the UL direction, wireless MM communications are generally asymmetric. These requirements lead to a 1/5 asymmetry factor between the UL and DL in the omnidirectional and tri-sectored BS antennas. The main improvement of tri-sectored frame corresponds to increase the throughput in the central cell, by a factor of N_{sec}. This N_{sec} increase occurs both in DL and UL, due to the use of a more favourable frame format.

Nevertheless, as resources are still needed for the BS-to-RS communication, some configurations with no relays, e.g., with tri-sectored BSs, may still lead to better efficiency in theoretical terms. If there was no coverage difficulties, topologies with no relays would consequently still have a higher throughput performance.

An additional challenge has been to optimize the energy saving when RSs are switched-off during either the night period or the weekends [3], when the traffic load is low [4]. In these periods, although the value for the transmitter power is kept the same the central coverage zone of the cell is zoomed out. During the night and weekends, the offered traffic significantly decreases and RSs may sleep whilst increasing the range of the central coverage zone of the cell. When a RS is working at the sleep mode, the air-conditioner and other energy consuming equipment can be switched-off. In this case, the coverage zones of the RSs in the sleep mode zooms in to 0 [3] and the central BS coverage zone zooms out to guarantee the coverage of the cell.

This special form of cell zooming may be explored to benefit from the lowest traffic demand and save power. The energy trade-offs arising from this process need therefore to be analyzed under simple assumptions for the energy consumption of each element of the BSs and RSs.

Cost/Revenue optimisation of the cellular planning was also a goal. Formulations have been proposed to take into account the interference in cellular coverage and reuse geometries, without and with the use of relays, in the Frequency Division Duplexing (FDD) mode. Optimisation of the cost/revenue trade-off provides a means of combining several contributing factors in cellular planning, including the determination of the reuse pattern, coverage distance, and the resulting supported throughput, following the vision proposed in [5]. This paper explores new methodologies to the optimisation of the fixed WiMAX network planning, finding efficient ways to reduce interference between co-channel cells, redesigning the structure of the frames, and optimising the system capacity and coverage.

The remainder of the paper is organised as follows. Section 2 addresses the impact of interference and MCSs into the planning process. The subframe structure is presented in Section 3, which also highlights its relation and differences in comparison with IEEE 802.16j. Section 4 presents aspects of the determination of the system capacity, including a brief description of the adopted formulation and results for the supported throughput. Green engineering aspects are discussed in Section 5, where a solution coping with cell zooming is proposed, where the coverage zone from the central BS is zoomed out while the coverage zone from the RSs is zoomed in to zero. Section 6 describes the cost/revenue model and discusses the optimisation results. A comparison is performed between the cases of absence and presence of cell zooming (with RSs switch-off during low traffic periods/empty hours). Finally, Section 7 presents the conclusions.

2 Impact of Interference and MCSs

In Fixed WiMAX, the supported physical user throughput is a function of the supported MCS, which in turn depends on the achievable CNIR compared with the minimum CNIR, $\text{CNIR}_{\min}$ for each MCS, as shown in Table 1 (where $\text{Auxfactor}(d)$ allows for computing the supported throughput as a function of d and the maximum supported throughput in the cell $R_b(0)$). It is therefore important to analyse the evolution of the CNIR against choices of several system parameters as well as the chosen co-channel reuse factor. To guarantee Fixed WiMAX with no coverage gaps near cell edges, the CNIR

Table 1 Auxiliar factor for the contribution of the different MCS in the communication between the RS and SSs.

ID	MCS	$\text{CNIR}_{\min}$ [dB]	Physical thr. [Mbps]	AuxFactor(d)
1	BPSK 1/2	3.3	1.41	1.41/5.64
2	BPSK 1/4	5.5	2.12	2.12/5.64
3	QPSK 1/2	6.5	2.82	2.82/5.64
4	QPSK 3/4	8.9	4.23	4.23/5.64
5	**16-QAM 1/2**	**12.2**	**5.64**	**1**
6	16-QAM 3/4	15.0	8.47	–
7	64-QAM 2/3	19.8	11.29	–
8	64-QAM 3/4	21.0	12.27	–

must be higher than 3.3 dB throughout the cell. This value corresponds to the $\text{CNIR}_{\min}$ in order to use BPSK 1/2 MCS. As FDD is used, analytical modelling of coverage and frequency reuse problems can only be carried out in Fixed WiMAX [6]. The approach accounts for carrier-to-noise and carrier-to-interference constraints [7]. The situation presents the distance associated with coverage and interference for a 2D geometry with six interferers at the first tier, when the mobile user is at a distance d from its serving BS [6].

The modified Friis propagation model is assumed at 3.5 GHz and the values of different parameters are considered as $P_t = -2$ dBW, $\gamma = 3$, in urban areas (no shadowing), $G_t = 17$ dBi, and $G_r = 9$ dBi for BS to SS and SS to BS [8], and $P_t = -2$ dBW, $\gamma = 3$, $G_t = 17$ dBi (for RS/SS communication), and $G_r = 28$ dBi for the RS (BS to RS and RS to BS). The difference between receiver gains for RS/BS communication and RS/SS (or BS/SS) communication is because, in the RS, we assume we may use a directional antenna, pointing directly towards the central BS; this antenna has a gain of ~ 28 dBi [9].

The radio frequency bandwidth, noise figure, and frequency are $b_{\text{rf}} = 3.5$ MHz, $N_f = 3$ dB, and $f = 3.5$ GHz [8], respectively. The worst-case interference scenario is considered, when the mobile unit is in the cell edge, where co-channel interference is higher. This worst-case DL scenario occurs when the BS of the serving cell transmits to the most distant possible location of subscriber station (SS) it is serving, using a channel (or sub-channel) on which the SS is also receiving interference from the BSs of the six co-channel hexagonal neighbouring co-cells. Note that, if D is the reuse distance, there are tiers of interference at distances D, $2D$, etc. However, if a high value for the propagation decay exponent is set, it is a valid approximation to only consider the first tier of interference [8]. For the UL, the worst-case scenario

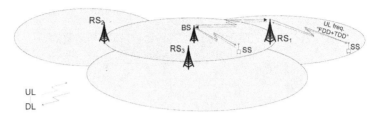

Figure 1 BS, RS and respective 'hexagonal' coverage areas.

occurs when the SS is transmitting to the BS from the cell edge, while inter-fering mobiles are on the boundary between interfering cells' edges and the serving cell of the SS. When a sectored BS antenna is considered the number of interfering cell is decreased, and system capacity increases. Details are given in [10, 11].

3 Sub-Frame Structure and IEEE 802.16j

A comparison of the correspondence between the throughput and the CNIR is performed for the RSs, BSs and SSs. In the considered multihop context, a cell is composed by the central coverage area, served by the BS, and three 240° sector coverage areas, served by individual RSs (RS_1, RS_2 and RS_3), as shown in Figure 1. While the BS antenna may be either omnidirectional or sectored (120° sectors) RS antennas for communication with BS are con-sidered to be directional (e.g., 120° sectored or narrower beamwidth ones), to reduce the received interference from BSs and facilitate non-overlapping coverage with the central zone of cell.

While the BS backhaul is assured in the usual terms for mobile commu-nications (e.g., cable or micro-wave radio link), RS backhauling is supported by using special specific sub-frames within the radius channel created for that purpose [12].

Our proposal on frames is inspired in the sub-frame structure from [13] and explores the inclusion of RS DL traffic/communications from RS to SS into the UL frequency sub-frame, differently from the proposal for IEEE 802.16j [14]. Another main difference between this proposal and IEEE 802.16j consists of only considering single-hop communications among the BS and RSSs, while IEEE 802.16j allows for multihop communications [15].

These assumptions for the frame are also inspired in the IEEE 802.16-2004 frames, which consists of two sub-frame, operate in FDD, DL and

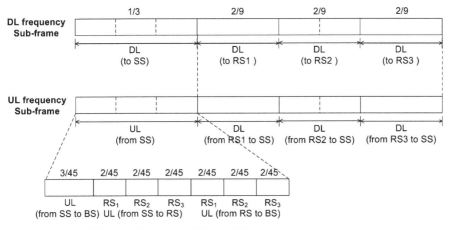

Figure 2   Structure of DL and UL frequency sub-frames.

UL transmitted at simultaneously. Although the version of fixed WiMAX we consider here originally used FDD, this proposal implies that Time Division Duplexing (TDD) needs to be additionally supported (over the FDD frame structure) for RS-to-SS communications, as shown in Figure 1. Besides, the proposal for DL and UL frequency sub-frames from Figure 2 (omnidirectional BS antenna case) assumes an asymmetry factor of 1:5 between the UL and DL. This type of RS is not standardised and available yet but this structure for frequency sub-frames is flexible enough to accommodate changes in the relay topology (e.g., facilitating the inclusion of mobile RSs), as RSs and SSs already incorporate TDD in the UL frequency sub-frame. The advantage of using relays arises from the fact the co-channel interference now comes from cells at a larger distance [11, 16].

The duration of each sub-frame may be 5 ms; this information is given by 'Alvarion', the manufacturer of the communications equipment that has been used during this research [17, 18]. Note, however, that there may be some similarities between the sub-frame structure proposed in this work and the frame with transparent relaying in the 802.16j standard. With transparent relaying, the RSs do not forward framing information; hence do not increase the coverage area of the wireless access system; the main use of this mode is to facilitate capacity increases within the BS coverage area. This type of relay is of lower complexity, and only operates in a centralised scheduling mode and for topology up to two hops. This mode assumes that the RSs have some small buffering capability, such that multiple hops via the relay can be scheduled in different frames. For example, data can be transmitted from the BS to the RS in one frame, and the same data can be forwarded from the RS to the SS in the subsequent frame.

For the cells with relays, the frame structure in the case of tri-sectored BS is different from the previous one, as proposed in [10, 11]. The main improvement of this tri-sectored frame corresponds to the increase of the throughput in the central cell by a factor of the number of sectors, N_{sec}, as there is a carrier assigned to each sector. This N_{sec} increase takes place both in DL and UL, due to the use of a more favourable frame format.

4 System Capacity

4.1 Formulation for the Physical and Supported Throughput

The formulation for the throughput is the one from [5, 16]. However, a formulation, proposed in [11], and adapted to topologies with RSs, is followed here. As presented in the previous section, the frames need to guarantee enough resources for BS-to-SS communications but also for BS-to-RS and RS-to-SS communications. Worst-case situations between the BS-to-RS and RS-to-SS communications are considered. These formulations are based on the dependence of the physical throughput on CNIR for different MCSs and are proposed in [10], as well as the algorithm for the computation of the throughput (implemented in MATLAB).

Different topologies may be considered to calculate the CNIR, corresponding to worst-case situations on the edge of the cell, where higher co-channel interference takes place, due to the proximity between cells. Results were presented in [10] for DL and UL geometries, using omnidirectional and tri-sectored BS antenna (applying also sub-channelisation). From these CNIR experimental results, one may conclude that for the communication between BS and RS for the DL (RS-to-BS for UL) one obtains the highest values for CNIR, followed by the communication between BS and SS for DL (SS-to-BS for UL), and the communication between RS and SS for DL (SS-to-RS for UL). The higher the reuse pattern, K, is the higher CNIR is.

There is a correspondence between the values of CNIR and the physical throughput, $R_{b[Mb/s]}$. An example is presented in Figure 3 for a configuration with relays. The right hand side curves show the correspondence between the curves of CNIR and the throughput. The stepwise behaviour comes from the correspondence between $CNIR_{min}$, in dB, and the physical throughput for each MCS.

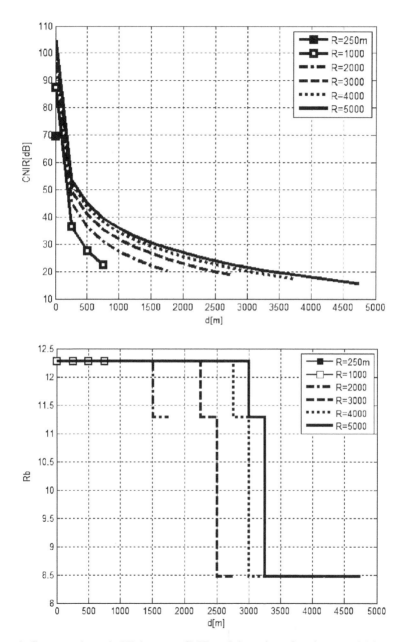

Figure 3 Correspondence in UL between CNIR and throughput for tri-sectored BS antennas and sub-channelisation for $K = 3$.

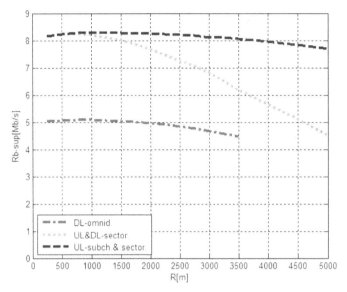

Figure 4   Supported cell/sector throughput vs. *R* for $K = 3$ (no relays).

4.2 Results in the Absence and Presence of Relays

By considering the formulation for the supported throughput from [5, 16], the curves for the supported throughput versus distance may be obtained for different values of K. Results for the cell/sector supported throughput are shown in Figure 4 for $K = 3$ and the absence of relays, and in Figure 5 for the case of the DL and presence of relays.

For the former, different cellular configurations, with omnidirectional or tri-sectored BS antennas, are considered, and the use of subchannelisation may be considered in the UL.

Some of the curves with no subchannelisation are either impossible to obtain at all or after a given R because the physical throughput near the cell edge reaches 0 Mb/s, and full cell coverage may not be guaranteed. Achievable results for the supported throughput (with tri-sectored BS antennas and $K = 1$) are of the order of 4.5 Mb/s, as shown in [5]. For the latter case (presence of relays), a tri-sectored BS antenna is considered and the case of the DL with $K = 3$ is analyzed in Figure 5. Owing to the availability of three times of the resources of the BS, we may conclude that using a tri-sectored BS antenna is clearly advantageous, compared with the omnidirectional case (where achievable values for the supported throughput are of the order of

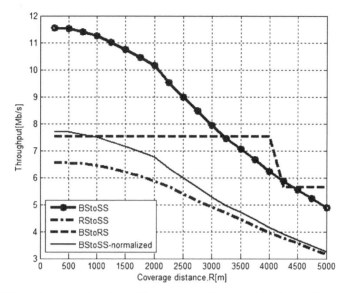

Figure 5 Throughput as a function of the coverage distance with relays and sectored cells in the DL, $K = 3$.

2 Mb/s [10] against 6.5–7.5 Mb/s with tri-sectored cells). Although the curves are not presented here, for $K = 1$, the supported throughput is of the order of 1.1 Mb/s for omnidirectional cells against 3.6 Mb/s with tri-sectored cells [10]. In the omnidirectional case, only if three transceivers are made available in the omnidirectional BS the results for the throughput become similar.

4.3 Equivalent Supported Throughput

With the proposed frame format presented, communications using a given frequency carrier are only from/to a sector and a RS. Hence, to obtain the supported throughput, the contribution from the central cell results from multiplying the sector supported throughput by N_{sec}. The equivalent supported throughput in a hexagonal coverage zone (or cell) with an area of $(3\sqrt{3}/2)\cdot R^2$ is therefore given by

$$
(R_{b-\text{sup}})_{\text{equiv}} = \frac{R_{b-\text{tot}}}{3} = \frac{N_{\text{sec}} \cdot R_{b-\text{central}} + 3 \cdot R_{b-\text{RS}-\text{zone}}}{3}
$$

$$
= \frac{1}{2} \cdot N_{\text{sec}} \cdot R_{b-\text{central}-\text{norm}} + R_{b-\text{RS}-\text{zone}} \tag{1}
$$

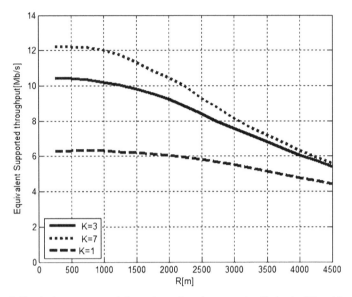

Figure 6 Equivalent supported throughput for tri-sectored cells in the DL with relays.

where $R_{b-\text{tot}}$ is the total throughput in the multihop cell (formed by the central zone plus RS zones). The use of sectored cells corresponds to an N_{sec} increase in both DL and UL traffic from/to the BS, due to the use of a more favourable frame format, as proposed in [10]. Curves shows the average throughput for $K = 1, 3$ and 7. Figure 6 shows the equivalent supported throughput for the DL communication using tri-sectored BS antennas.

The equivalent supported throughput is used in Section 6 to calculate the costs, revenues and profits.

5 Cell Zooming with Relay Stations Switch-off

According to Niu et al. [3], when a BS/RS is working in the sleep mode, the air conditioning devices and other energy consuming equipment may be switched-off. BS/RS sleeping may significantly reduce the energy consumption of the WiMAX cellular network. In the solution we propose in this paper the three RS coverage zone working in the sleep mode zooms in to 0 while its central BS coverage zone zoom out to guarantee the coverage, as shown in Figure 7. The coverage radius for the zoomed out cell is given by $R_{z-\text{out}} = \sqrt{3}R'$, where R' is the radius for the BS/RS 'hexagonal' coverage zones from the cell with relays.

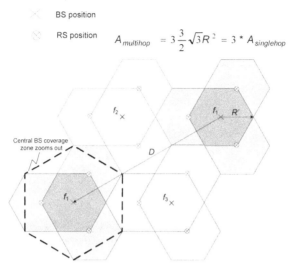

Figure 7   When RSs go to sleep mode the central coverage zone zooms out.

It is nevertheless worthwhile to note that, in comparison with this 'zoomed out' central coverage zone, the topology with RSs enables us (i) to achieve a more regular coverage whilst guaranteeing almost regular physical layer throughput along wider zones of the cell (both central BS and RSs coverage zones) and (ii) to guarantee Line-of-Sight (LoS) coverage zones throughout the whole area, as shadowing is more efficiently avoided through the use of four stations (one BS and three RSs).

Results for the supported throughput are presented in Figure 8. When the RSs are switched-off, if the frame format needs to be kept there will be a partial loss of capacity (the part of the sub-frame dedicated to the communication with the RSs is being wasted). As a consequence, although the total throughput is obtained by multiplying the cell/sector throughput by three (because there are three available carriers, in the omnidirectional case, and three sectors in the 'zoomed out' cell with one carrier each, in the tri-sectored case), one still needs to consider the effect of the DL sub-frame format in the resulting supported throughput, i.e., a factor of 1/3 in both cases [11], yielding to an overall multiplying factor of 1. Note that, in Figure 8, there are different horizontal axis for the cells with relays (R' varies from 0 to 2886.8 m in this case) and for the ones with zoomed-out central coverage zone and no relays ($R_{z-\text{out}}$ varies from 0 to 5000 m).

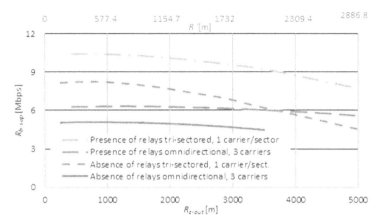

Figure 8 Comparison of the equivalent supported throughput between the cells with relays and the zoomed-out cells (if the frame format is not adaptively adapted in the absence of relays) and the cells with relays.

Figure 9 presents the results for the throughput in the case the frame format can be adaptively adapted; hence, the factor 1/3 is not applied anymore in the absence of relays. Note however that in [11, section V.E.], the comparison between the tri-sectored BS for the topology with the presence and the absence of relays assumes one carrier per sector but erroneously fails to multiply the sector throughput by the number of sectors, N_{sec}, in the absence of relays. Hence, the economic performance in the tri-sectored case and absence of relays should be approximately three times higher than the erroneously represented in [11, figure 18]. Instead, the true behaviour is in line with the one discussed in Section 6.1.

This improvement leads to an advantage for the topologies with no relays that may possibly compensate the better (and more regular) coverage achieved in topologies with relays. However, it is not reflected in the results for cell zooming from this paper yet, as we assume it is not possible, in practice, to adaptively change the frame format during the empty hours by now (as the mobile terminals that support communication with relays are not flexible enough to allow for sub-frame format changes).

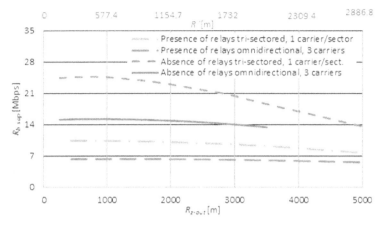

Figure 9 Equivalent supported throughput for the cells with relays and the zoomed-out cells (if the frame format may be adaptively adapted in the absence of relays).

6 Cost/Revenue Optimisation

6.1 Comparison between the Absence and Presence of Relay Stations

The optimisation of the cost/revenue trade-off provides a means of combining several contributing factors in WiMAX cellular planning: determination of the reuse pattern, coverage distance, and the resulting supported physical throughput. The cost/revenue function takes into account the cost of building and maintaining the fixed WiMAX infrastructure, and the way the number of channels available in each cell affects operators' and service providers' revenues. Fixed costs for licensing and spectrum bandwidth auctions should also be taken into account. The economic analysis is referred as a cost/revenue performance analysis. Although considers project duration of five years as a working hypothesis in radio and network planning, it is decided to analyze costs and revenues on an annual basis. The analysis is under the assumption of a null discount rate. By no means is it intended to perform a complete economic study in this paper, e.g., via the computation of the net present value; the aim is simply to present initial contributions that facilitate the incorporation of the main cellular planning optimisation aspects into the economic analysis. Appropriate refinements would be needed to perform a complete economic analysis based on discounted cash flows, e.g., to compute the net present value. Furthermore, the aim is to apply the optimisation model from [10, 11] to facilitate WiMAX cellular planning. A similar investigation was followed in [19] for hierarchical WiMAX-WiFi networks but it is not followed here. Instead, the approach from [5] is followed here.

The cost per unit area is given by [8]

$$C_{(\mathrm{\euro}/\mathrm{km}^2)} = C_{f(\mathrm{\euro}/\mathrm{km}^2)} + C_b \cdot N_{\mathrm{hex}/\mathrm{km}^2} \tag{2}$$

where C_{fi} is the fixed term of the costs, and C_b is the cost per BS assuming that only one transceiver is used per cell/sector. In the multi-hop case, with relays the number of hexagonal coverage zones per unit area is given by

$$N_{\mathrm{hex}/\mathrm{km}^2} = \frac{2}{3 \cdot \sqrt{3}R'^2} \tag{3}$$

and the cost per BS is given by

$$C_b = \frac{C_{\mathrm{BS}} + C_{\mathrm{bh}} + C_{\mathrm{ins}}}{N_{\mathrm{year}}} + C_{\mathrm{M\&O}} \tag{4}$$

where N_{year} is the project's lifetime (assumed to be $N_{\mathrm{year}} = 5$), C_{BS} is the cost of the BS, C_{bh} is the cost for the normal backhaul, C_{inst} is the cost of the installation of the BS, and $C_{\mathrm{M\&O}}$ is the cost of maintenance and operation [10].

In our formulation, as the supported throughput was obtained for an hexagon-shaped coverage zone (whose area is $(3\sqrt{3}/2) \cdot R'^2$), we maintain the formulation from [5] replacing cells by hexagon-shaped coverage zones, and $N_{\mathrm{hex}/\mathrm{km}^2} = N_{\mathrm{cell}/\mathrm{km}^2} \cdot 3$. Note that the three RS coverage zones exactly correspond to an area of two hexagons. Besides, note that the value for C_{BS} is such that the cost of the BS and the RSs (1/5 of the cost of the BS) are averaged in a way it enables to obtain the value for the cost of an 'equivalent BS' for each of the three coverage zones, i.e., $C_{\mathrm{BS-equiv.}} = (C_{\mathrm{BS}} + 3 \cdot C_{\mathrm{RS}})/3$. As only the central BS needs a fixed backhaul, C_{bh} is one third of the value for a normal BS. Besides, as one needs to install one BS and three RSs, the installation cost (for this 'equivalent BS') is 4/3 the cost of a normal BS. It is assumed that the operation and maintenance (M&O) costs of the RSs are half the value of the ones for the BS, such that $C_{\mathrm{M\&O-equiv \cdot BS}} = (C_{\mathrm{M\&O-BS}} + 3/2 \cdot C_{\mathrm{M\&O-BS}})/3$.

The revenue in a hexagonal-shaped coverage zone per year, $(R_v)_{\mathrm{cov\_zone}}$, can be obtained as a function of the equivalent supported throughput per coverage zone, $R_{b-\mathrm{sup[kbps]}}$, and the revenue of a channel with a data rate $R_{b[\mathrm{kbps}]}$, $R_{b[\mathrm{\euro}/\mathrm{min}]}$, by

$$(R_v)_{\mathrm{cov-zone}} = \frac{N_{\mathrm{hex}/\mathrm{km}^2} R_{(b-\mathrm{sup})\mathrm{equiv}} \cdot T_{\mathrm{bh}} \cdot R_{R_b}[\mathrm{\euro}/\mathrm{MB}]}{R_{b-\mathrm{ch[kbps]}}} \tag{5}$$

Table 2 Costs with relays with different antennas and $K = 1$ (one carrier per cell/sector); for different values of K and different number of carriers the value of C_{fi} needs to be changed accordingly while the values for the other parameters remains the same.

Costs	Omnidirectional	Tri-sectored
$C_{fi[€/km^2]}$	15.63	47.14
$C_{BS[€]}$	7680	6800
$C_{inst[€]}$	1333.33	2000
$C_{bh[€]}$	833.33	833.33
$C_{M\&O[€/year]}$	833.33	833.33

where $R_{(b-sup)equiv}$ is fixed by Equation 1. T_{bh} is the equivalent duration of busy hours per day, and R_{b-ch} is the bit rate of the basic 'channel'. In the tri-sectored case, one assumes that each sector has one different transceiver. Furthermore, there is a separate frequency channel available for each sector.

The revenue per unit length or area per year, $Rv[€/km^2]$, is obtained by multiplying the revenue per cell by the number of cells per unit length or area. The profit, in absolute and percentage terms, was defined according to Velez et al. [5].

According to the assumptions with relays from [10, 11], the cost parameters from Table 2 were considered for $K = 1$. The value of the fixed cost is 'per carrier'. For different values of K, the fixed cost, C_{fi}, increases proportionally to K while the values for the other parameters keep being the the same [10]. For example, for $K = 3$, it becomes $C_{fi} = 3 \cdot 3 \cdot 15.63 = 140.68$ €/km^2 (with three carriers) in the omnidirectional case, and $C_{fi} = 3 \cdot 47.14 = 140.68$ €/km^2 in the tri-sectored case.

As a bandwidth of 31.5 MHz may be available for an operator, it is worthwhile to compare the case of tri-sectored cells (or central coverage zones, if the topology is with relays) and $K = 3$, with the case $K = 3$ with omnidirectional BS antenna getting three carriers, and the situation without RSs in both tri-sectored an omnidirectional antenna cases from [5]. In this situation, as in the $K = 1$ situation, the number of carriers and the supported throughput are multiplied by three.

It should be noted that, with sectored cells, the cost of the frequency carriers licence (C_{fi}) with $K = 3$ is three times the cost for the licence with omnidirectional BS antenna and $K = 3$, as $K \cdot N_{sec} = 9$ carriers need to be available. Besides, when more than one frequency carrier is considered per cell, extra channel equipment (transceivers) needs to be added to the BS (or RS) rack [20]. We assume a 60% increase on the cost of BS and RS equipment if tri-sectored antennas and RF equipment (including the outdoor units, ODUs) are considered. This means we assume that the channel equipment costs are 30% of the BS (or RS); hence, with tri-sectored equipment, two times 30% needs to be added to the cost. For $K = 3$, with 3 frequency carriers and omnidirectional BS antennas, although C_{BS}, C_{inst}, C_{bh} and $C_{M\&O}$ keep being the same, as one considers $C_{BS-omni} = 14400$ €and $C_{RS} = 2880$ €then one obtains $C_{BS-equivalent} = 7680$ €. For the tri-sectored case, one considers $C_{BS-tri} = 15000$ €and $C_{RS} = 1800$ €(one assumes the RS is cheaper because it is simpler), yielding $C_{BS-equivalent} = 6800$ €.

In Figure 10 we represent the coverage distances for the coverage zones with RSs by R' while $R = \sqrt{3}R'$ is the coverage distance for a cell with no RS whose area is the same (compared with the area of the cell with a central coverage zone plus three RS coverage zones). With no RSs and tri-sectored central coverage zone (sect.&no RSs) the economic performance would be weak (see Figure 10, example for $R_b = 0.005$ €/MB) if only one carrier may be used (as erroneously presented in [11, section V.E]). In this paper, owing to the proper accounting of the contribution from the three sectors (see results for the supported throughput in Figure 9), the profit in percentage with tri-sectored BS and no RSs achieves values ~2000–2500% for R up to 1400 m, an important change compared with [11, figure 18]. With omnidirectional BS antenna, the profit in percentage is ~1400–1500% up to 1400 m. With tri-sectored BS and RSs the profit is also higher than the one obtained for the omnidirectional case (~900–1000% for R' up to 800 m). Note that the costs of the BS and the three RSs are accounted for all together.

With omnidirectional BSs and no RSs (omni.&no RSs), under the same total bandwidth, three carriers may be used and the profit in percentage varies between ~1500 and 1200% for coverage distances (R) lower than 1400 m, Figure 10. With RSs and omnidirectional antennas in the BS, profits of the order of 800–900% are achievable for R' up to 1000 m [11].

6.2 Economic and Environmental Impact of Cell Zooming

We assume the values from Table 3 for the power of the BS and RS equipment, whose reference values are partially extracted from [21]. The values for the power consumption of the BS were chosen based on the powers for the Alvarion BS equipment while the values for the power consumption of the RS equipment refer to the powers of the micro-BS Alvarion equipment (the comparison is done because, as the RS, it can also be connected to two ODUs). Each BS sector has a different ODU, whose power consumption is 40 W each. The RSs will have an ODU for the communication with the RS

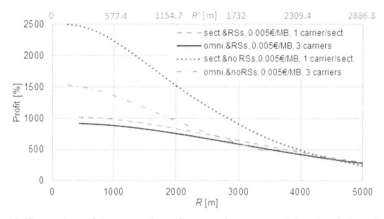

Figure 10 Comparison of the economic performance between omnidirectional (3 carriers) and tri-sectored (one carrier/sector) BSs in the presence and absence of relays under the same total BW for price $R_{144} = 0.005$ €/MB, in the DL and $K = 3$.

Table 3 Power consumption parameters for the BSs and RSs.

Station	BS		RS
	Tri-sectored	Omni.	
Power for the full chassis [W]	420		80
Number of sectors	3	1	–
Power for the outdoor unit(s) [W]	120	40	80
Total power of the BS/RS equipment alone [W]	540	460	160
Power consumption for the router/switch [W]	100		–
Power consumption for the ventilator [W]	40		20
Total power consumption for the stations [W]	680	600	180
Annual energy consumption [kW·h]	6000	5250	1750

and a different one for the communication with the SSs (40 + 40 = 80 W total).

The power consumption for the fan of the cooler ventilation system is assumed to be 40 W for the BS equipment and 20 W for the RS equipment. Besides, we assume the power consumption for the switch/router at the BS is 100 W (and there is no such switch/router at the RS shelter). As a consequence, the total power consumption values for the stations are the following ones: $P_{\text{BS-tri}} = 540+100+40 = 680$ W, $P_{\text{BS-omni}} = 460+100+40 = 600$ W and $P_{\text{RS}} = 160 + 20 = 180$ W. From this analysis, one may conclude that, by itself, the use of RSs instead of full functionality BSs lead to circa 70% reduction in the power consumption for their coverage zones.

These RSs can be switched-off in periods when the traffic exchange is low. In a scenario where RSs are zoomed in to zero during the night periods and weekends, by switching the RS equipment off, and the central BS coverage zone is zoomed out, leading to a coverage distance of $R_{z-\text{out}} = \sqrt{3}R'$, the total power becomes now simply the power of the central BS (either 680 or 600 W, for tri-sectored and omnidirectional BSs, respectively). In the full functionality cell with RSs the total power is $680 + 3 \cdot 180 = 1220$ W or $600 + 3 \cdot 180 = 1140$ W, respectively. This is approximately twice the power of the zoomed out cell. The 540 W reduction on the power corresponds to a given reduction in operations costs, proportional to the time period the RSs remain switched-off.

During the whole year, the total energy waste in RSs is $24 \cdot 365 \cdot 540 = 4730.4$ kW·h. If the price of the energy is 0.10 €/kW·h the electricity cost is 473.04 €/year. If the RSs are switched-off overnight (for eight hours each night during the working days) and during the while weekend (48 hours) then the total period when the energy is saved is $5 \cdot 8 + 2 \cdot 24 = 88$ hours (against 80 hours of full functionality cell operation), i.e., full operation lasts only for $80/168 = 47.6\%$ of the time. Therefore, by switching-off the three RSs of each cell the economic annual expenditure resulting from the power reduction in each cell is $473.04[€] \cdot 0.476 = 225.17$ €/year per cell, corresponding to a reduction in the annual cost per cell of 247.17 €/year.

The aforementioned reduction in the cost per cell corresponds to a reduction of the operation costs of the 'equivalent BS' of $247.17/3 = 82.62$ €/year (approximately 10% of the operation and maintenance cost).

As we assume the DL sub-frame format cannot be changed (to a more favourable one) when the RSs are switched-off, the economic performance is the one presented in Figure 11 (example for $R_b = 0.005$ €/MB). Note that the ~83 €/year reduction in the operation and maintenance costs are reflected in the computations for the zoomed out central BS coverage zone cell (in the no RSs case).

As the throughput decreases with no RSs (see results in Figure 8) the economic performance is lower. However, it is important to highlight that in the absence of RSs, in the case of the zoomed out central BS coverage zone (with these RSs in the sleeping mode and its cooling system switched-off) the economic performance is reasonable (700–800% and 400–450% profit up to $R = 1$ km with tri-sectored and ominidirectional BSs, respectively) compared with the case of the full cell functionality (~1000% and ~900% profit, respectively). Besides, the switch-off of the RSs as the clear advantage of the power saving, and yields an important economic impact.

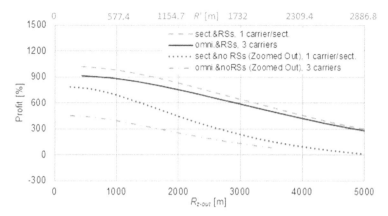

Figure 11 Comparison of the economic performance between omnidirectional (3 carriers) and tri-sectored (one carrier/sector) BSs in the presence of relays and with the central BS coverage zone zoomed out (while RSs coverage zoom in to zero) under the same total BW for price $R_{144} = 0.005$ €/MB, in the DL and $K = 3$.

If adaptive radio is possible in WiMAX and the frame format can be changed when RSs are switched-off, the economic performance will be closer to the one presented in Figure 10 (although the reduction in the maintenance and operation cost arising from it were not fully incorporated in the analysis in this figure).

Further work is needed to analyze the trade-offs between the clear economic advantage (as well as the advantage in the supported throughput) and the resulting loss in the coverage. With only one central BS the 'illumination' throughout the zoomed out cell may not be as complete as the one with one from the central BS plus three RSs. From this point of view, omnidirectional cells should be avoided as they will only support the lowest order MCS near the cell edge (both in topologies with the presence and absence of RSs). The use of tri-sectored antennas is therefore preferable. For example, with tri-sectored BS antennas, the lowest order MCS is

- QPSK 1/2 (ID $= 3$ and $(C/N)_{min} = 5.5$ dB) with no RS ($R_{z-out} = \sqrt{3} \cdot 1750 = 3031$ m);
- QPSK 3/4 (ID $= 4$ and $(C/N)_{min} = 8.9$ dB) with RSs (for $R' = 1750$ m).

As $(C/N)_{min} = 3.3$ dB for the lowest order MCS in Fixed WiMAX (BPSK 1/2), in the absence of relays, there is a difference of only 2.2 dB between the actual threshold for the MCS at the cell edge and the threshold enabling a non-null throughput (against a difference of 5.6 dB with relays). These difficulties need to be properly addressed in the future.

7 Conclusions

Frequency reuse topologies have been explored for 2D broadband wireless access topologies in the absence and presence of relays, and the basic limits for system capacity and cost/revenue optimisation have been discussed.

For a given coverage area, throughput is a stepwise function that decreases as distance from the base station increases. Its value depends on the supported MCS for each coverage ring. In this paper, the supported throughput has been computed for cellular WiMAX topologies, with deployed relays, by weighting the available throughput at each coverage ring with the area (or size) of the coverage area ring. Throughput typically decreases as the cell radius increases, although through the use of subchannelisation it is possible to keep its value steady at least up to a cell radius of 5000 m. With the use of sectored cells, the supported throughput is higher, corresponding to the selection of the highest order MCSs. However, as tri-sectored equipment is more expensive and there is a need for three times more bandwidth to be provided to the BS in this case, costs are also higher.

Cellular deployment with relays can be cheaper than using BS alone. Because the use of relays (and a structure was proposed for the sub-frames to guarantee resources for BS-to-SS communication as well as BS-to-RS and RS-to-SS communication) to help on improving coverage while mitigating interference, may lead to lower costs, it is worthwhile to analyse the impact of using them on costs and revenues. WiMAX cost-benefit optimisation has been explored in this paper for the case where relays are used. Although the reuse distance is augmented by a factor of $\sqrt{3}$, it was first shown that, with omnidirectional BSs, the use of relays corresponds to lower values of the supported throughput for $K = 3$. It was also verified that the presence of subchannelisation in the UL only improves the results for the highest values of R. Only the consideration of tri-sectored BS antennas with $K = 3$ (at the cost of extra channels, where nine channels corresponds to a bandwidth of 31.5 MHz) obtains values of system throughput comparable (although lower) to the those without using relays. This is due to the more favourable frame format that is employed under the use of tri-sectored BS antennas.

With no RSs and omnidirectional BSs ('omni.&no RSs') with $K = 3$, under the same total bandwidth, three carriers may be used. The profit in percentage terms varies between $\sim$ 400 and 300% for coverage distances lower than 1400 m (one assume a price per MB of 0.005 €/MB). However, with tri-sectored BSs ('sect.&noRSs'), as the throughput is multiplied by $N_{sec} = 3$, it achieves values of ~2000–2500% for R up to 1400 m. With RSs, the use of tri-sectored BSs (sect.&RSs) is not advantageous relatively to the 'no RS' case, as the profit decreases down to ~900–1000% (for R up to 1000 m).

To save energy during empty traffic periods, cell zooming may be applied in conjunction with relays going into sleep mode at times of low load. As we assume the DL sub-frame format cannot be changed (to a more favourable one) when the RSs are switched-off, the economic performance is better with RSs. With no RSs, as the throughput decreases, the economic performance is lower. However, it is important to highlight that, if RSs go into sleep mode (and their cooling system is switched-off), the economic performance of the zoomed out cell is still reasonable (for tri-sectored and ominidirectional BSs, 700–800% and 400–450% respectively profit up to $R = 1$ km) compared with the case where RSs are deployed (~1000% and ~900% profit, respectively).

If adaptive radio is possible in WiMAX and the frame format can be changed when RSs are switched-off, the economic performance will be superior. However, the resulting loss in the coverage with no relays has not been properly addressed yet. With only one central BS the 'illumination' throughout the zoomed out cell may not be as complete as the one with one from the central BS plus three RSs.

Acknowledgments

This work was funded by 'Projecto de Re-equipamento Científico REEQ/1201/EEI/ 2005, UbiquiMesh, OPPORTUNISTIC-CR, COST IC 0905 'TERRA', COST 2100, by the Marie Curie Intra-European Fellowship OPTIMOBILE (FP7-PEOPLE-2007-2-1-IEF), by the Marie Curie Reintegration Grant PLANOPTI (FP7-PEOPLE-2009-RG), and partially supported by the ICT-ACROPOLIS Network of Excellence, FP7 project number 257626, www.ict-acropolis.eu.

References

[1] IEEE Std 802.16-2009 (Revision of IEEE Std 802.16-2004), IEEE standard for Local and metropolitan area networks – part 16: air Interface for fixed broadband wireless access systems 3, The Institute of Electrical and Electronics Engineers, New York, USA, 2009.

[2] P.R. Adry and M.A.H. Dempster. *Introduction to Optimisation Methods*. Chapman and Hall, London, UK, 1974.

[3] Zhisheng Niu, Yiqun Wu, Jie Gong and Zexi Yang, 'Cell zooming for cost-efficient green cellular networks. *IEEE Communications Magazine*, 48(11):74–79, November 2010.

[4] L.M. Correia, D. Zeller, O. Blume, D. Ferling, Y. Jading, I. Goídor, G. Auer and L. Van Der Perre. Challenges and enabling technologies for energy aware mobile radio networks. *IEEE Communications Magazine*, 48(11):66–72, November 2010.

[5] Fernando J. Velez, A. Hamid Aghvami and Oliver Holland. Basic limits for fixed WiMAX optimization based in economic aspects. *IET Communications*, Special Issue on WiMAX Integrated Communications, 4(9):1116–1129, June 2010.

[6] Ramjee Prasad and Fernando J. Velez. *WiMAX Networks: Techno-Economic Vision and Challenges*. Springer, Dordrecht, the Netherlands, 2010.

[7] Georg Bauer, Ranjan Bose and Rolf Jakoby. Three-dimensional interference investigations for LMDS networks using an urban database. *IEEE Transactions on Antennas and Propagation*, 53(8):2464–2470, August 2005.

[8] Pedro Sebastião, Fernando Velez, Rui Costa, Daniel Robalo and António Rodrigues. Planning and deployment of WiMAX networks. *Wireless Personal Communications*, 55(3):305–323, November 2010.

[9] Fernando J. Velez, Rui Costa, Daniel Robalo, Marco Marques, Cláudio Comissário, José Riscado and Victor Cavaleiro. Design and installation of pre-WiMAX radio links and relays. In *Proceedings of the 11th International Symposium on Wireless Personal Multimedia Communications (WPMC 2008)*, Lapland, Finland, September 2008.

[10] Maria del Camino Noguera. Cost/revenue optimization of cellular planning for fixed and portable WiMAX networks with relays. Final Year Project, Universidade da Beira interior, Covilhã, Portugal, July 2010.

[11] Fernando J. Velez, M. Kashif Nazir, A. Hamid Aghvami, Oliver Holland and Daniel Robalo. Cost/revenue trade-off in the optimization of fixed WiMAX deployment with relays. *IEEE Transactions on Vehicular Technology*, 60(1):298–312, January 2011.

[12] Jeffrey G. Andrews, Arunabha Ghosh and Rias Muhamed. *Fundamentals of WiMAX – Understanding Broadband Wireless Networking*. Prentice Hall, Upper Saddle River, NJ, USA, 2007.

[13] Christian Hoymann, Karsten Klagges and Marc Schinnenburg. Multi-hop communication in relay enhanced IEEE 802.16 networks. In *Proceedings of the 17th IEEE International Symposium on Personal, Indoor and Mobile Radio Communications (PIMRC 2006)*, Helsinki, Finland, September 2006.

[14] IEEE Draft Standard P802.16j/D5. Part 16: Air interface for fixed and mobile broadband wireless access systems – Multihop relay specification. The Institute of Electrical and Electronics Engineers, New York, NY, USA, May 2008.

[15] Vasken Genc, Sean Murphy, Yang Yu and John Murphy. IEEE 802.16j Relay_based wireless access networks: An iverview. *IEEE Wireless Communications Magazine*, 15(5):56–63, October 2008.

[16] Fernando J. Velez, M. Kashif Nazir, A. Hamid Aghvami, Oliver Holland and Daniel Robalo. System capacity. In Ramjee Prasad and Fernando J. Velez (Eds.), *WiMAX Networks: Techno-Economic Vision and Challenges*. Springer, Dordrecht, the Netherlands, 2010.

[17] BreezeMAX 3000 Technical Specification, Release 2.5. Visited 2010.

[18] Raj Jain, Chahchai So-In and Abdel-Karim al Tamimi. System-level modelling of IEEE 802.16e mobile WiMAX networks: Key issues. *IEEE Wireless Communications Magazine*, 15(5):73–79, October 2008.
[19] M. Ibrahim, K. Khawam, A.E. Samhat and S. Tohme. Analytical framework for dimensioning hierarchical WiMAX-WiFi networks. *Computer Networks*, 53(3):299–309, 2009.
[20] Kwang-Cheng Chen and J. Roberto B. de Marca. *Mobile WiMAX*. John Wiley and Sons/IEEE Press, Chichester, West Sussex, UK, 2008.
[21] Alvarion. *BreezeMAX Micro Base Station System Manual*, S/W Version 1.5, Alvarion, Tel Aviv, Israel, April 2005.

Biographies

Fernando J. Velez (M'93-SM'05) received the Licenciado, M.Sc. and Ph.D. degrees in Electrical and Computer Engineering from Instituto Superior Tecnico, Technical University of Lisbon in 1993, 1996 and 2001, respectively. Since 1995 he has been with the Department of Electromechanical Engineering of Universidade da Beira Interior, Covilhã, Portugal, where he is Assistant Professor. He is also a researcher at Instituto de Telecomunicações, Lisbon, and was a Marie Curie Research Fellow at King's College London in 2008/09. He made and still makes part of the teams of RACE/MBS, ACTS/SAMBA, COST 259, COST 273, COST 290, IST-SEACORN, IST-UNITE, OPTIMOBILE, PLANOPTI, COST 2100, COST IC0902 and COST IC0905 'TERRA' European projects, he participated in SEMENTE, SMART-CLOTHING and UBIQUIMESH Portuguese projects, and he was or is the coordinator of five Portuguese projects: SAMURAI, MULTIPLAN, CROSSNET, MobileMAN and OPPORTUNISTIC-CR. He is the coordinator of the WG2 (on Cognitive Radio/Software Defined Radio Coexistence Studies) of COST IC0905 'TERRA'. He is also acting as the IEEE VTS European Chapter coordinator since 2010. Professor Velez has authored two books, ten book chapters, more than 100 papers and communications in international journals and conferences, plus 25 in national conferences, is a senior member of IEEE and Ordem dos Engenheiros (EUREL), and a member of IET and IAENG. His main research areas are cellular planning tools, traffic from mobility, MAC and routing protocols, cross-layer design, spectrum sharing/aggregation, and cost/revenue performance of advanced mobile communication systems.

Maria del Camino Noguera obtained her MSc degree in Telecommunication Engineering at Miguel Hernandez University of Elche (UMH), Elche,

Spain, in 2010. Her MSc project entitled 'Cost/Revenue optimization of cellular planning for fixed and portable WiMAX networks with relays' was developed at Instituto de Telecomunicações, Universidade da Beira Interior, Covilhã, Portugal. She is currently a Global Customer Experience Engineer at Hewlett-Packard, Iberia. The main tasks on her position are administration, management and troubleshooting of customer environments, providing solutions to customers regarding Vmware, Hp-UX and Linux technologies. Maria has also co-authored the WPMC 2010 paper: 'Basic limits for system capacity and cost/revenue optimisation: A formulation for fixed WiMAX'.

Oliver Holland obtained his B.Sc. degree (with First Class Honours) from Cardiff University, and his Ph.D. from King's College London. He is working within the ICT-ACROPOLIS Network of Excellence on Dynamic Spectrum Access (DSA) solutions and is part of the management team of that project, and is also contributing to the UK's Virtual Centre of Excellence in Mobile and Personal Communications (Mobile VCE) on DSA techniques for Green Radio. Oliver is Treasurer of the IEEE DySPAN Standards Committee (DySPAN-SC); he is also a member of the IEEE P1900.6 and IEEE P1900.1 working groups, was a Technical Editor of the IEEE 1900.4 standard, and is Technical Editor for the developing IEEE 1900.1a standard. He is a member of the Management Committee representing the UK within two prestigious collaborative 'COST' actions on the topic of cognitive radio, and holds various leadership positions within these COST actions. Oliver has served on the Technical Programme Committees of all major conferences in the area of mobile and wireless communications, has served as Session Chair and Panellist at a number of conferences covering Green Radio and Cognitive Radio, among other topics, and frequently serves as a reviewer for various prestigious international conferences and journals. He was guest editor of the special issue 'Achievements and the Road Ahead: The First Decade of Cognitive Radio', which appeared in *IEEE Transactions on Vehicular Technology*, was co-chair of the 'Cognitive Radio and Cooperative Communications' track of IEEE VTC 2010-Fall, and he is an Associate Editor of *IEEE Transactions on Vehicular Technology*. He is an Officer of the IEEE Technical Committee on Cognitive Networks (TCCN), serving as liaison between TCCN and COST IC0905 'TERRA', and between TCCN and DySPAN-SC, and he is currently the Chair of the United Kingdom and Republic of Ireland Chapter of the IEEE Vehicular Technology Society. Oliver has jointly authored over 90 publications on a variety of topics, including several book chapters and one patent. The 68 of his publications that Google Scholar locates have been cited more than 290 times.

A. Hamid Aghvami (M'87-SM'91-F'05) received his M.Sc. and Ph.D. degrees from the University of London, London, U.K., in 1978 and 1981, respectively. In 1984, he joined the academic staff of King's College London, where he was promoted to Reader in 1989, became a Professor of telecommunications engineering in 1993, and is currently the Director of the Centre for Telecommunications Research. He carries out consulting work on digital radio communications systems for both British and international companies. He is the author of more than 500 technical papers and has given invited talks on various aspects of personal and mobile radio communications and courses on the subject worldwide. Professor Aghvami is a Fellow of the Royal Academy of Engineering and the Institution of Electrical Engineers. From 2001 to 2003, he was a member of the Board of Governors of the IEEE Communications Society. He is a Distinguished Lecturer of the IEEE Communications Society and has been a member, Chairman, and Vice Chairman of the technical program and organising committees of several international conferences. He is also the Founder of the International Conference on Personal, Indoor, and Mobile Radio Communications.

Introducing Energy Awareness in the Cognitive Management of Future Networks

Kostas Tsagkaris, George Athanasiou, Marios Logothetis, Yiouli Kritikou, Dimitrios Karvounas and Panagiotis Demestichas

Department of Digital Systems, University of Piraeus, 18534 Piraeus, Greece; e-mail: {ktsagk, athanas, mlogothe, kritikou, dkarvoyn, pdemest}@unipi.gr

Received 25 June 2011; Accepted: 4 July 2011

Abstract

The current circumstances on a worldwide level urgently impose to exploit technology in order to reduce environmental pollution, CO_2. emissions and waste. The current technologies and the provisioned evolution steps take into consideration these facts and contribute to achieve greener footprint. This paper describes technologies as important elements in the design of Energy-aware Future Networks. They comprise Energy-aware Opportunistic Networks and Traffic Engineering schemes that can be seen as two major extensions towards future networks in the wireless infrastructure-less and wired backhaul/core segments, respectively. In parallel, the role of Cognitive Management Systems for enhancing these technologies with intelligent features that can assist in the optimization of network performance goals, including green targets, is also pointed out. Several simulation results evince how the proposed schemes can contribute in achieving greener footprint in the context of Future Networks.

Keywords: cognitive management, energy-aware, green footprint, opportunistic networks, traffic engineering, future networks.

Journal of Green Engineering, 383–412.

1 Introduction

Networking systems and user devices have become in the past decade an integral tool of people every day lives; in personal professional and leisure activities. Therefore, it is essential to evolve not only the devices themselves, but also the networks, in order to meet both people needs with respect to applications, as well as to the way and the quality of provisioning of these applications for the users. Consequently, certain technological requirements emerge; Personalization, context awareness, always best connectivity, ubiquitous service provision and seamless mobility are some of the high priority requirements [1–4]. Most importantly, current socio-economic circumstances in Europe and worldwide impose immediate actions with respect to achieving pollution reduction, environmental-friendly behaviour and adaptation to every aspect of peoples' routine [5, 6]. To this end, green aspects must be considered towards the evolution of the networking solutions so as to satisfying today's needs while preparing for tomorrow, future networks.

Obviously, addressing such requirements and ever increasing complexity with the goal to select the ideal operating state of networks, is a very difficult task to achieve, considering the huge number of controllable parameters and different network performance objectives. Cognitive Management Systems (CMSs) have been proposed as a promising technology towards this direction. In general, CMSs are characterized by their ability to empower networks with advanced, intelligent processing and decision making e.g., based on learning and reasoning so as to dynamically adapt to varying network conditions in order to optimize performance.

Framed within the above, in this paper we advocate that Energy-aware Opportunistic Networks and Traffic Engineering can be seen as two major extensions towards future networks in the wireless access and wired/core segments, respectively. At the same time they render a fruitful landscape for naturally evolving the Cognitive Management Systems (CMSs) developed as part of the cognitive research findings within the FP7 European project End-to-End Efficiency (E^3) [1] and most importantly, further elaborated and specified in the Reconfigurable Radio Systems (RRS) Technical Committee [15] of ETSI standardization body.

More specifically, the OneFIT [20] research project has recently proposed and started working on a solution that comprises Opportunistic Networks (ONs), CMSs and control channels. Differentiating to what has been described so far [7], ONs can be seen here as temporary extensions to the infrastructure, which are dynamically built, based on connectivity opportunities and by exploiting flexible spectrum management [1] and ad-hoc networking technologies. Four basic technical challenges need to be addressed with respect to these ONs; the determination of the suitability of the appropriate circumstances to proceed with their creation, their creation per se, the maintenance of the offerings that they were created for and their release, as long as they have fulfilled their goal. In this context, the paper describes the five technical scenarios related to ONs that are used in [20] so as to leverage the arising challenges and the evolved management systems that need to be developed for addressing them. In addition, we also demonstrate how the management decisions made by these cognitive systems can result in higher green footprint, mainly in terms of lower electrical energy consumption (lower transmission powers,) and less investments in and accordingly deployment of hardware.

In addition, the idea of ONs and the QoS-demanding applications that will need to support, unavoidably leads to more traffic that must be served by the infrastructure-based backhaul/core network. This also leads to increased power consumption and complexity in terms of required configuration/management complexity. Therefore, it is essential to reconsider the design and the management of this part of Future Networks, as well. An important goal in this direction is to achieve the best ratio of performance to energy consumption and at the same time assure manageability. To this effect, an Energy-Aware Traffic Engineering (ETE) scheme is proposed for the core/backhaul segments of a future network, providing balanced, congestion free, energy-aware and operator governed network operation. Once again, it is envisaged that mixing such schemes with CMSs and self-x capabilities will also empower Future Networks with the capability to adapt their behavior in an autonomous manner using learning and knowledge sharing.

Accordingly, the rest of this paper is structured as follows: Section 2 focuses in the need for Cognitive Management systems and their role in the emerging wireless world through the prism of ETSI RRS. Section 3 focuses on the OneFIT solution that is based on ONs, describes the tackled scenarios and shows how the latter can be exploited so as to increase energy-awareness in future networks. Section 4 complements the puzzle by discussing challenges and proposing energy-aware schemes related to the infrastructure-based core/backhaul parts of the network. Finally the paper is concluded in Section 5.

2 Cognitive Management Systems

As already stated, CMSs have the ability to empower networks with advanced, intelligent processing and decision making. Particularly CMSs incorporate self-management and learning mechanisms in order to overcome the complexity of the infrastructure and the wireless access [8].

Self-management enables a system to identify opportunities for improving its performance and adapting its operation without the need for human intervention. Learning mechanisms are important so as to increase the reliability of decision making. They also enable proactive handling of problematic situations, i.e. identifying and handling issues that could undermine the performance of the system before these actually occur.

Generally a CMS enables a system to identify opportunities for improving its performance and adapting its operation without the need for human intervention. CMSs make and enforce decisions by taking into account the context of operation (environment requirements and characteristics), goals and policies, profiles (of applications, devices and users), and machine learning (for managing and exploiting knowledge and experience). Learning mechanisms are important so as to increase the reliability of decision making. They also enable proactive handling of problematic situations, i.e. identifying and handling issues that could undermine the performance of the system before these actually occur.

Actually, there has been a lot of research in the field of cognitive networks and their management; it spans physical layer [9–11], network layer [12] and application layers [13, 14]. The FP7/ ICT E^3 project [1] also worked towards integrating cognitive wireless systems in the Beyond 3G (B3G) world, evolving current heterogeneous wireless system infrastructures into an integrated, scalable and efficiently managed B3G cognitive system framework. The delivered result comprises a set of entities that exhibit cognitive functionality and interfaces for introducing cognition in the wireless world. In addition and more importantly, the ETSI RRS TC [15] delineated the standardisation roadmap of these functional entities and interfaces as a hallmark certifying their timeliness and importance for emerging networks. A graphical representation of the current view of the wireless world as formed by ETSI TC RRS is given in Figure 1. In this figure, the Cognitive Control Network (CCN) on the one part and the Composite Wireless Network (CWN) on the other part, need to collaborate in order to efficiently provide the requested applications/services to both emerging (multiradio) and legacy user devices. As far as CCN is concerned, the management relies on autonomic/cognitive

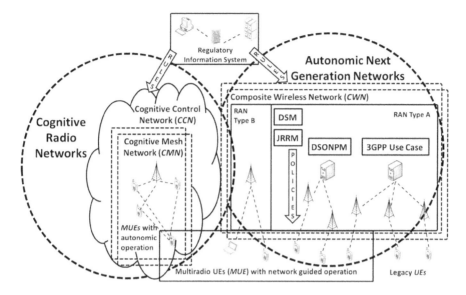

Figure 1 Emerging wireless world as per ETSI RRS view [19].

elements, operator governance through policies, as well as on protocols so as to achieve cooperation between the CCN and with the CWN.

Challenges arising with respect to the above include:

- Potentials for efficient FI application provisioning.
- Improved resource utilisation and "green footprins" with respect to re-duced costs (Capital Expenditures – CAPEX, Operational Expenditures - OPEX, total cost of ownership).
- Dynamic spectrum management, ad-hoc network operation.
- Standardization activities (evolved ETSI TR102.682 [16], ETSI TR102.683 [17], IEEE Std 1900.4-2009 [18]).
- Coordination with CWN.

On the other hand, the characteristics of CWNs are the following:

- They comprise a set of radio networks, heterogeneous or not.
- Each CWN is operated by a single Network Operator (NO).
- The network management system is common for all the radio networks in CWN.

Particularly, CWNs' management relies on a set of specified func-tional entities, namely 3GPP Self Organizing Network (SON) (self-management/planning, 3GPP use cases), JRRM (Joint Radio Resource Management), DSONPM (Dynamic Self-Organized Network Planning and Management) and DSM/FSM (Dynamic/Flexible Spectrum Management) [15]. JRRM is an entity that enables management of composite radio resources and selection of radio access technologies for user traffic connections. DSM provides long and medium term recommendations for the (technically and economically) available amount of spectrum introducing flexible spectrum management scheme. Finally, DSONPM caters for the medium and long term management decision of reconfigurable network segments, realizing the management domain.

The challenges also arising for CWN include:

- QoE/QoS, cost efficiency (OPEX, CAPEX).
- End-to-end perspective: evolution, intelligence embodiment, federation for end-to-end optimality.
- Efficient validation (simulation, prototyping, experiments, trials, pilots).

Consequently, based on the emerging wireless world (ETSI RRS view), the proposed scheme with ONs [20] can be seen as a solution to address challenges appearing in CCN, while Traffic Engineering can resolve problems arising in the area of CWN [21].

Despite the extended research that has been done in the field of cognitive management technologies, it is necessary to further evolve the aforementioned concepts. This means that they need to be adjusted to the current needs of users, as well as to the needs imposed by the society as a whole. As mentioned before, the need to protect the environment and investigate ways to consume less energy and create environment friendly technologies has emerged, more compelling than ever. The following sections present the current technology evolution in these research fields, highlighting their green footprint perspective.

3 Opportunistic Networks

3.1 The Idea of Opportunistic Networks

ONs have been defined in [20] as coordinated extensions of the infrastructure networks and they are operator-governed as far as resources management, policies, and information/knowledge are concerned. They are dynamically created based on the operators' spectrum/ policies/ information/ knowledge, in places and times that efficient service provisioning to mobile users is needed. They can comprise network elements of the infrastructure as well

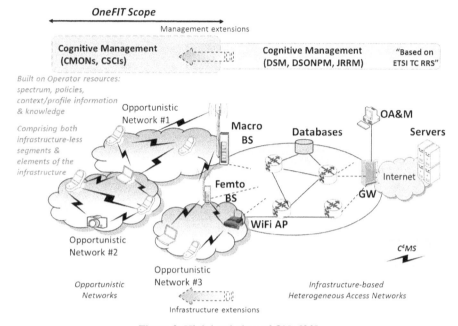

Figure 2 High level view of ONs [20].

as terminals/ devices, potentially organized in an infrastructure less (ad-hoc) mode and they are created and "live" for a particular time interval that needed for setting up and providing QoS demanding applications (Video Streaming, VoIP, IPTV, etc.) to users in the most efficient manner.

As an extension to ETSI RRS specified CMSs described above, two types of systems are envisaged, called "Cognitive systems for Managing the Opportunistic Network" (CMONs) and "Cognitive management Systems for Coordinating the Infrastructure" (CSCIs). The main idea in the aforementioned schemes is to provide the means to facilitate close cooperation between the infrastructure and the ONs, as depicted in Figure 2. Such collaboration is essential for ensuring viability, deployment and value creation for all the stakeholders. In addition, the "Control Channels for the Cooperation of the Cognitive Management System" (C4MS) is introduced in order to coordinate the functionality of the previous entities.

In this context, five technical scenarios are considered and related to the management of ONs. They are used to describe the arising challenges (including the green footprint) which will be addressed by the development of

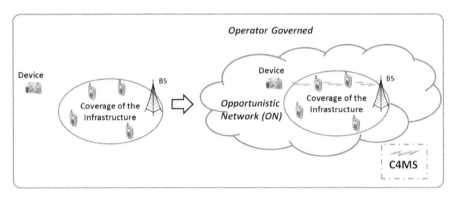

Figure 3 Scenario 1: Opportunistic coverage extension.

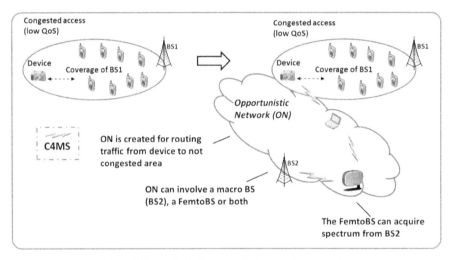

Figure 4 Scenario 2: Opportunistic capacity extension.

cognitive management systems as part of the ongoing work in this effort. The scenarios are as follows:

1. Opportunistic coverage extension (Figure 3).
2. Opportunistic capacity extension (Figure 4).
3. Infrastructure supported opportunistic ad-hoc networking (Figure 5).
4. Opportunistic traffic aggregation in the radio access network (Figure 6).
5. Opportunistic resource aggregation in the backhaul network (Figure 7).

In the following subsection the above-mentioned scenarios are described and the green footprint of each scenario is presented, accordingly.

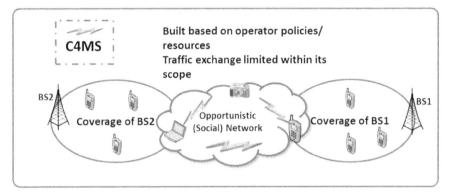

Figure 5 Scenario 3: Infrastructure supported opportunistic ad-hoc networking.

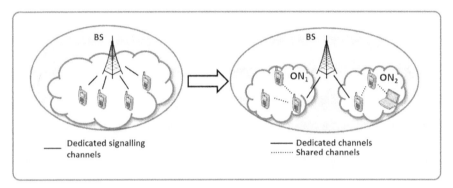

Figure 6 Scenario 4: Opportunistic traffic aggregation in the radio access network.

3.2 Green Footprint of ONs

In this subsection, the five scenarios are presented in more detail, depicting the different facets of the ON-based solution along with its potential for contributing in a "greener" footprint.

1. Opportunistic coverage extension
In this scenario the ONs are used for enabling the devices to communicate over infrastructure networks, even if there is no direct connection to an infrastructure network. This may be occurring as the user's device supports the air interface of the infrastructure, but is out of its coverage or has bad coverage. Another reason is that the user's device may be in the coverage of

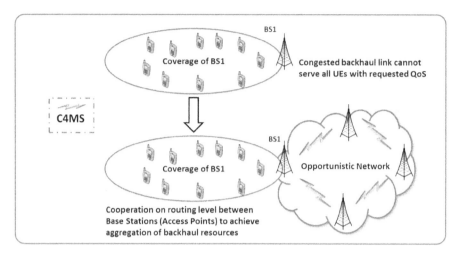

Figure 7 Scenario 5: Opportunistic resource aggregation in the backhaul network.

the infrastructure network, but does not support the air interface provided by it.

In this scenario lower transmission power levels are achieved, which leads to lower electrical energy consumption. Therefore, a higher green footprint is achieved that is also reflected to lower OPEX and particularly to the reduction of the expenses made by the operator for the operation of the infrastructure.

2. Opportunistic capacity extension

In this scenario, ONs are used to resolve the capacity/congestion issues in mobile (infrastructure) networks. In other words, the ON is used in order to redirect the access route and avoid connecting to a congested network infrastructure with questionable offered QoS levels.

In this scenario the claim that the ONs influence the green footprint is strengthened, as they contribute to the reduction of the transmission power and consequently lead to lower electrical energy waste. Higher bit-rates are also possible, while capacity extension leads to less investment in infrastructure and consequently less hardware deployed. This means that lower OPEX, as well as CAPEX are achieved.

3. Infrastructure supported opportunistic ad-hoc networking

ONs are also used along with the local Peer-to-Peer (P2P) communications paradigm, so as to enable the optimization of resource usage and the provision of new services in a localized manner. The ON created is completely infrastructure-less, but still operator-governed through the provision of resources and policies. The rationale is to exploit the fact that often the end-points of an application are physically close devices at any given time (e.g., attendees to a conference or concert, travellers in the same bus or train etc.) so that traffic exchange can be limited within its scope.

The green footprint of this scenario is also proved by the energy consumption diminishment that is achieved through the localization of application provisioning. Higher bit rates are possible, as well.

4. Opportunistic traffic aggregation in the Radio Access Network
In this case the ONs are used for enabling the optimization of resource usage and QoS provision in the Radio Access Network (RAN). This is achieved by "forcing" a limited sub-set of the ON terminals to exchange data with the infrastructure; these terminals aggregate/ distribute data from/ to all the other terminals in the ON. This situation improves the degree of traffic aggregation and caching, which is useful for the overall network performance improvement.

Obviously, in this case the green footprint is achieved by succeeding to support limited ON terminals, fact that leads to lower electrical energy consumption.

5. Opportunistic resource aggregation in the backhaul network
Lastly, the ONs and multipath routing are used for enabling the optimization of backhaul resource usage in the infrastructure network. In this case, the ON is created over access points rather than user terminals. It thus offers a new focus on system performance improvement.

In this scenario, capacity extension leads to less investment in infrastructure and consequently less hardware deployed, which consequently results to higher green footprint and lower CAPEX.

3.3 Performance Evaluation

This section discusses on the simulations we have conducted for two of the aforementioned scenarios in order to investigate the green benefits and the overall network performance from the creation of the ON. We will also study performance metrics in order to assure that the achievement of greener footprint does not negatively affect the overall network efficiency in the application provisioning.

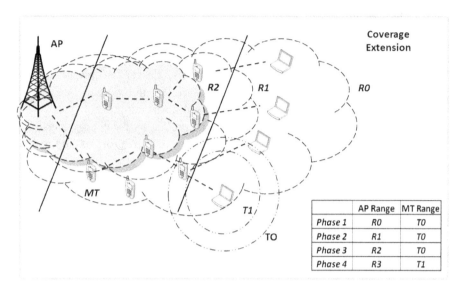

	AP Range	MT Range
Phase 1	R0	T0
Phase 2	R1	T0
Phase 3	R2	T0
Phase 4	R3	T1

Figure 8 Simulation test cases.

3.3.1 Test Case 1 – Coverage Extension

A set of test cases were executed in the simulation environment, which was based on the widely used NS-2 simulator [24] and ran on an Intel Core i5 2.3 GHz with 4 GB of RAM and a 64-bit Operating System.

Without loss of generality, the topology comprises a single AP supporting IEEE 802.11 g technology with a maximum offering data rate at 54 Mbps. A set of 12 mobile terminals (MTs) are supported within the range of the AP, the four of which are selected to be the application consumers. VoIP application, based on the G.711 [25] voice encoding scheme for both the caller and the callee, is considered in the simulation test cases exhibiting stringent resource requirements and real time sensitivity.

Describing the test cases depicted in Figure 8, four phases (steps) are considered, each one corresponding to a specific percentage of the initial TRx power of the AP/MTs, namely: 100% (initial)/100% (initial), 80%/100%, 60%/100% and 60%/60%, thus resulting in ranges R0/T0, R1/T0, R2/T0 and R2/T1, respectively. In general, during the reduction of the AP's TRx power, some of MTs are left out of the APs' range. These MTs are then supposed to create ONs with intermediate MTs in an ad-hoc manner and operate in WLAN 802.11g, as well. In particular, the initial transmission power of the AP and MTs is set equal to 0.03 W and 0.02 W, respectively.

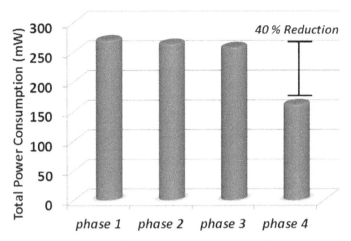

Figure 9 Total power consumption in mW.

Furthermore, each phase evolves also sub-phases depending on the mobility level of the intermediate MTs that are inside a predefined mobility domain using a random waypoint mobility model. We assumed 7 mobility levels (0 m/sec–15 m/sec), with the same maximum speed for all the MTs that are inside this domain and pause times equal to 1 sec. Finally, for completion reasons, we also experiment with the routing protocols [26] namely, DSR, AODV, OLSR and GRP, which will be used to route traffic to MTs that are found out of range during the AP's and MTs' transmission power reduction.

Figure 9 depicts the total power consumption that is required for supporting the data traffic in the test case prior to (phase 1) and after the formation of the ON (phase 2–4). All the nodes in the network and the infrastructure element (AP) are considered in the computation of the total energy consumption. As depicted, the formation of the ON can result in a reduction of 40% of the initial transmission power. This result supports our initial claims of better use of resources in terms of energy consumption.

In the sequel, we also focus on specific QoS metric, which is used to evaluate conditions and assist in coming up with useful recommendations with respect to the creation of the ONs networks with the possible green gains. We focus herewith on performance metric associated with the QoS levels that the applications will be provided through the ON(s), namely Application Delay (sec).

Figure 10 depicts the end-to-end delay that VoIP suffers averaged on the application MTs. The single dotted line corresponds to the maximum accept-

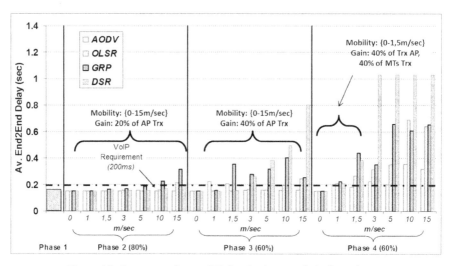

Figure 10 Average end-to-end Delay (sec) per node in four phases.

able delay. Generally, as the mobility level increases, the overall delay also increases. This is due to the fact that the mobility in the intermediate nodes, can significantly impact the performance of the ad-hoc routing protocols, including the packet delivery ratio, the control overhead and the data packet delay [27].

Moreover as the number of intermediate nodes increases, while the AP's range is shrinking, the overall delay also increases since more MTs participate in routing and forwarding of the received packets. In the same figure, the existed solutions in terms of mobility level are depicted with the anticipated green benefits. In phase 2 and 3, it is observed that all mobility levels has acceptable values and can result to a 20 and 40% reduction of transmission power, respectively.

On the other hand in phase 4 there are only three acceptable solutions (0–1.5 m/sec) and can result in a reduction of 40% of the required transmission power. Therefore, there is some degree of freedom regarding the creation of the ON to be applied, which can vary depending on the level of emphasis given to specific target QoS levels and aimed savings in transmission power.

In general, as simulations showed, AP/MTs transmission power reductions of 60% can be obtained without impacting too much the service provisioning. This means that the supported application remains at acceptable QoS levels with less AP/MT power resources. Therefore this reduction will result important savings in the total transmission power in the network.

3.3.2 Test Case 2 – Opportunistic Traffic Aggregation in the Radio Access Network

Focusing on the traffic aggregation scenario described above, there may be users that face poor channel quality towards the infrastructure, because they may residing at the edge of the AP and at the same time very good channel quality towards some of their neighbours. It is obvious that users with poor channel quality, compared to those with better quality, need more resources (e.g., power, time) to transmit the same amount of data. After the creation of the ON, users with good channel conditions towards the infrastructure will be responsible for forwarding traffic to those that have poor channel conditions, through their direct interfaces. Therefore, the ON will increase the overall system capacity and resource utilization, and offer a service in an energy efficient manner.

For the simulations, a set of four nodes set-up direct connections (via cellular interfaces) with a network in order to transmit data packets of the size of 1 MB each. It is assumed that users' devices are equipped with 3G interfaces (for the connection with the AP) and with IEEE 802.11g interfaces for the peer-to-peer connections among them. At some point in time the quality of the nodes' connections significantly drops, thus the connection throughput is limited for three of them to 0.5 Mbps. At the same time, these nodes maintain very good channel quality towards some of their neighbours, offering a rate of 54 Mbps by using IEEE 802.11g interface. The AP in collaboration with the nodes, detects that situation, and initiates the process for the creation of an ON. They jointly determine one or several nodes, with high channel conditions to aggregate and/or relay traffic of other users, which have poor channel conditions towards the infrastructure.

Figure 11, depicts the anticipated average delivery latency prior to and after the formation of ON. It corresponds to the one-way time (in seconds) from the source sending a packet to the destination receiving it. With direct links, it is observed that the average delivery latency is around 13 sec, while the deployment of the ON yields a significant drop of this metric to 2.3 sec.

Moreover, Figure 12 depicts the total power consumption that is required for the traffic of the test case prior and after the creation of the ON. It considers again all nodes in the range of the AP and the infrastructure element. As Figure 12 depicts, the creation of the ON can result in a reduction of 22% of the required transmission power, which can be justified by the shorter direct links that are used for forwarding traffic within the ON. This result in this test case also proves our claims of better use of resources in terms of energy consumption. Finally, the CMSs can ensure fast and reliable establishment of

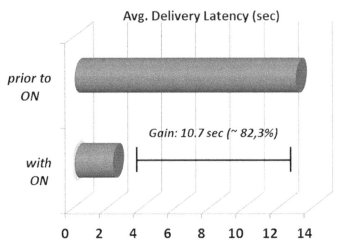

Figure 11 Average delivery latency estimation in sec.

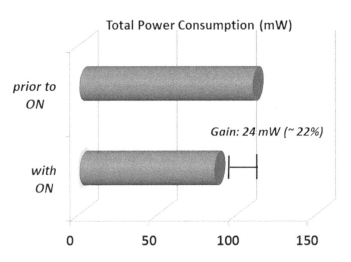

Figure 12 Total power consumption in mW.

ONs and perform well when facing same situations, thus resulting in faster reductions of the energy consumption, achieving efficiently green targets.

4 Infrastructure Networks

4.1 Future Core/Backhaul Networks

As mentioned before, the current network infrastructures face problems in keeping up with the requirements of their growing ecosystem and increased QoS demanding wireless /mobile access segment, mainly due to the incapability of their management systems to deal with current challenges. An efficient management system would require operators to be able to manage and to control their networks both effectively (reducing human intervention whilst optimizing resource usage, reducing costs through energy-efficient solutions, etc.) and flexibly.

However, typical management systems are designed in a bit-centric fashion offering reasonably stable bandwidth pipes to their customers, whereas the demands of today and tomorrow call for a service centric fashion which puts a strong focus on end-user satisfaction and energy efficiency, too. Currently, Operators and ISPs are far from being able to respond to the aforementioned demands since management and operational costs represent the majority of the total cost of ownership of networks, permitting only a limited amount of investment into new infrastructure and facilities.

One of the main characteristics in the era of Future Networks will be the growth of QoS-demanding applications that need to be supported. Unavoidably, this leads to increased traffic that has to be served by the deployed networks.

Figure 13 depicts the expected growth of traffic that has to be supported by the Future Networks in order to provide efficient service provisioning [22]. In addition, this also leads to increased power consumption and configuration/management complexity.

Recently, due to the increased energy prices, the growth of costumer population and the expanding number of services being offered by operators and ISPs, the energy efficiency issue has become a high-priority objective for the Future Networks. The continuously rising demands in network energy consumption essentially depend on new services that must be supported by the future infrastructures. Figure 14 depicts the Global e-Sustainability Initiative (GeSI) report [23]: In 2002, network infrastructures for mobile communication and for wired narrowband access caused the most considerable greenhouse contributions, since each of them weighs for more than 40% upon the overall network carbon footprint. The estimation for 2020 says that mobile communication infrastructures will represent more than 50% of network CO_2 emissions.

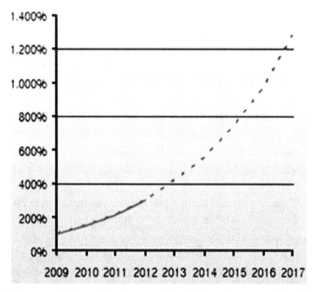

Figure 13 Traffic growth. Cisco visual networking index – forecast and methodology [22].

4.2 Green Footprint of Core/Backhaul Networks

The concept of "Future Internet Networks" is globally emerging as a federation research theme with the objective of overcoming the structural and cost limitations of the telecommunication infrastructures (mainly at the core level) and their management systems. Using Future Internet systems, Operators and ISPs should be able to manage their ever more pervasive and sophisticated networks, enabling:

- Dynamic, efficient and scalable support of a multiplicity of applications across federated administrative and technology domains.
- Light operations and migration to cost effective, secured, and manageable networking functionality.
- Autonomic management procedures in order to achieve the best ratio of performance to energy consumption and assure manageability.

Focusing basically on the last two objectives that are related to the green footprint of the Future Core/Backhaul Networks, we must highlight that given the high heterogeneity of networks and technologies, architectures, and operational constraints of protocols applied at different layers, the most efficient way to develop novel energy saving mechanisms is to concentrate on specific scenarios, investigate their demands on energy saving and design

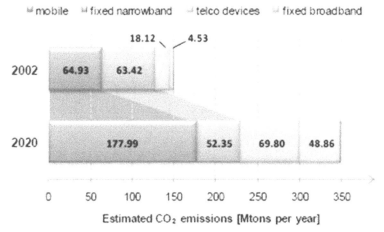

Figure 14 Global e-Sustainability Initiative (GeSI), SMART 2020: Enabling the low carbon economy in the information age [23].

specific energy-efficient protocols. Thus, the researchers must try to find specific solutions/mechanisms that will have negligible impact on the network level performance: *Energy-efficient router operation and switch architectures must be concerned. Moreover, new approaches must be investigated that will provide efficient and energy-aware network operation through sophisticated traffic engineering mechanisms. These energy-efficient traffic engineering schemes must allow the operators to balance the load and avoid failures, increasing in this way the reliability and improving the network performance.*

4.2.1 Green Traffic Engineering

Following up on our previous discussion we focus on traffic engineering and investigate ways of introducing energy-awareness in the network. Traffic engineering receives huge attention as one of the most important mechanism seeking to optimize network performance and traffic delivery. Wang et al. [28] gave an overview of the traffic engineering approaches that emerged the last years and placed focus on two major issues: quality of service (QoS) and network resilience. They provide a general classification of these traditional-objective traffic engineering approaches: intradomain vs. interdomain [29], MPLS-based vs. IP-based [30, 31], offline vs. online [32, 33], unicast vs. multicast [34, 35]. The work in this paper is inspired by these traditional traffic engineering approaches.

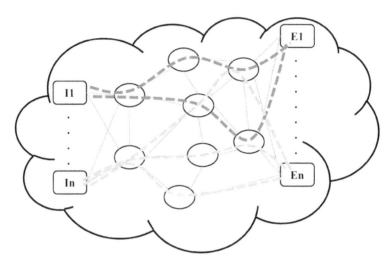

Figure 15 Example network topology.

A challenging task is to identify the main parts of the Internet that dominate its power consumption and investigate methods for improving energy consumption [36]. Moreover, the authors in [37] discuss the idea of dynamically turning part of the network operations into sleeping mode, during light utilization periods, in order to minimize the energy consumption. Recently, routing, rate adaptation and network control are mobilized towards energy-efficient network operation [38, 39]. Unfortunately, none of these approaches provide a general problem formulation in the direction of "coupling" the traditional traffic engineering objectives with the modern objectives (like energy-awareness). This paper is an attempt to "modernize" the research in this field.

We present below a distributed *Energy-Aware Traffic Engineering* (ETE) mechanism. We consider a network model, as depicted in Figure 15, where each ingress router may have traffic demands for a particular egress router or set of routers. We use multiple paths (MPLS tunnels) to deliver traffic from the ingress to the egress routers. We must mention here that traffic is split among the available paths at the granularity of a flow, to avoid reordering TCP packets or similar effects that lead to performance degradation (using efficient traffic splitting approaches, like [40]). In addition, we consider that the paths are computed and re-computed (if it is necessary) offline by the operator, since most of the operator's networks work in this way.

Table 1 Variables.

Variables	Description
L	Set of links in the network
IE	Set of Ingress to Egress node pairs
e_l	Energy consumption of the port connected to link l
P_i	Set of paths of Ingress to Egress node pair i
T_i	Traffic demand of Ingress to Egress node pair i
a_l	Binary variable: 0 if link l is sleeping, 1 if link l is active
u_l	Utilization of link l
c_l	Capacity of link l
x_{ip}	Fraction of traffic of Ingress to Egress node pair i, sent through the path p
r_{ip}	Traffic of Ingress to Egress node pair i, sent through path p
P_l	Set of paths that go through link l
L_i	Set of links that are crossed by the set of paths P_i
E	Demand of the operator in energy consumption

The main "cornerstones" in the proposed mechanism are the following *low-complexity* and *distributed* algorithms (Table 1 contains the definitions of the variables used):

- *Load Balancing*: Given the a_l values for the links in the network, find the corresponding x_{ip} values that provide balanced network operation in terms of link utilization. In order to provide an efficient solution we investigate for each ingress-egress node pair the paths that goes through the maximum utilized link. Then, we "relieve" this link by moving a portion of traffic Δx and provisioning it proportionally to the rest paths (inverse procedure of progressive filling that leads to optimal load balancing based on [41]). This procedure continues till convergence to the optimal x_{ip} values.

- *Energy Saving*: Given the x_{ip} values resulted from *Load Balancing*, find the maximum set of links that could be turned into sleeping mode. For each ingress-egress node pair we find the routers that are part of the active routes and turn the lines of their network card that are not used (by any path in the network) into sleeping mode.

The proposed approach (Figure 16) receives as input the operator request, as far as the energy consumption is concerned (E). Then, *Load Balancing* and *Energy Saving* are applied, by each ingress-egress node pair i in order to balance the link utilization in their paths and put the links that are not utilized into sleeping mode. Next, the new energy consumption level is compared to E in order to realize if we have reached the desired state. If not, the heuristic mechanism continues by excluding the path p with the minimum $x_{ip} T_i$ (light-

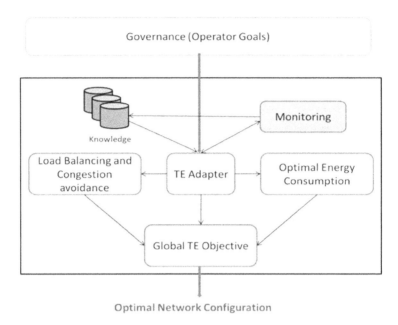

Figure 16 Cognitive/autonomic energy-aware traffic engineering.

est path). Traffic Engineering adapter controls the aforementioned procedure. The heuristic mechanism iterates based on the updated P_i values, optimizes x_{ip} and a_l values $\forall p \in P_i$, $l \in L_i$ and finally, stops when the operator's energy consumption goal is achieved.

We must highlight that ETE can be executed in an autonomous/cognitive manner using monitoring and knowledge sharing (Figure 16). In other words, the status of the system is continually monitored in order to apply ETE when needed. Moreover, knowledge (related to configuration actions and different states of the system) is stored for increasing reliability and automation of the system reactions. In this way there is no need for execution of the proposed heuristic mechanism when a "known" event happens in the network (e.g., new request with specific characteristics).

We present now the evaluation study of the proposed scheme. In order to provide realistic simulation results, we use real ISP topologies and traces provided by Rocketfuel tool [42]. In our simulation, we consider Tiscali (3257) traces and a network topology consisted of 18 routers and 77 links. We compare the performance of ETE to OSPF-TE [43] that was applied in Tiscali network when the traces were collected.

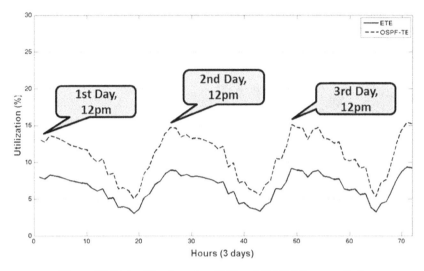

Figure 17 Link utilization when ETE and OSPF-TE are applied.

Figure 17 depicts the utilization of the links in the network when ETE and OSPF-TE are applied. We observe that ETE is able to keep the link utilization at low levels using the minmax link utilization policy that is adopted. On the other hand, OSPF-TE uses a dynamic procedure to calculate the link weights in order to route the traffic efficiently, which could lead to link overutilization.

Then, we plot the percentage of the initially consumed energy that is saved when ETE is applied. Similar to the previous test case, we consider Tiscali traces in order to build a relationship between the load of the traffic that must be supported in the network and the energy saving that could be achieved by ETE. Figure 18 visualizes that when the maximum link utilization is low, the energy saving is close to 50%. The percentage of saved energy continually drops while the traffic in the network grows and therefore the utilization of the links is becoming high.

Finally, Table 2 presents the existing tradeoff between the energy consumption and the maximum link utilization in the network. The first column contains the operator's request, as far as energy saving is concerned. In addition, in the next two columns we observe the percentage of the links that must be turned into sleeping mode and the routes that will be excluded in order to approach the corresponding E values. The last column presents the balanced link utilization that is achieved by ETE for each desired E level. It is obvious

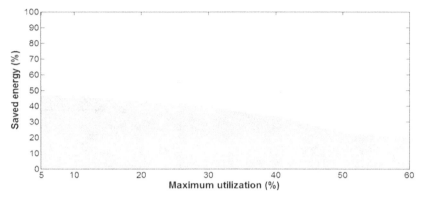

Figure 18　Percentage of saved energy vs. maximum link utilization.

Table 2　ETE performance – tradeoff.

Requested percentage for energy saving (E)	Percentage of "sleeping" links	Percentage of routes excluded	Maximum Maximum utilization
10%	5%	2%	6%
20%	18%	8%	13%
30%	24%	13%	21%
40%	36%	18%	42%
50%	45%	22%	58%

that there is an important tradeoff between the balanced and energy-aware network operation which is handled by ETE, based on the operator's goals.

5 Conclusions

In this paper we described several technologies envisioned as important elements in the design of Energy-aware Future Networks. Energy-aware Opportunistic Networks and Traffic Engineering schemes are presented as two major extensions towards Future Networks in the direction of introducing energy-awareness in the operation of wireless infrastructure-less and wired backhaul/core segments, respectively. Moreover, the role of Cognitive Management Systems for enhancing these technologies with intelligent features is also investigated in the paper. The simulation results depict the greener footprint that is achieved in the context of Future Networks by the proposed approaches. Future directions include: extended cognitive/autonomous functionality enhanced with learning and autonomic features and implementation/deployment using commodity hardware.

Acknowledgements

This work is performed in the framework of the European-Union funded project OneFIT (www.ict-onefit.eu). The project is supported by the European Community's Seventh Framework Program (FP7). The views expressed in this document do not necessarily represent the views of the complete consortium. The Community is not liable for any use that may be made of the information contained herein. Also the research leading to these results has been performed within the UniverSelf project (www.univerself-project.eu) and received funding from the European Community's Seventh Framework Programme (FP7/2007-2013) under grant agreement No. 257513.

References

[1] E^3 Project, http://www.ict-e3.eu
[2] P. Demestichas. Introducing cognitive systems in the wireless B3G world: Motivations and basic engineering challenges. *Telematics and Informatics Journal*, 27:256–268, February 2010, doi: 10.1016/j.tele.2009.08.002.
[3] V. Stavroulaki, Y. Kritikou and P. Demestichas. Introducing cognition in the management of equipment in the future wireless world. In *Proceedings of 19th IEEE International Symposium on Personal Indoor Mobile Radio Communications 2008 (PIMRC 2008)*, Cannes, France, September 2008.
[4] K. Tsagkaris, M. Logothetis and P. Demestichas. Studies on the potentials of the exploitation of infrastructure-less segments by composite wireless networks. In *Proceedings of OpnetWork 2010*, Washington, USA, August 30–September 2, 2010.
[5] G. Gür and F. Alagöz. Green wireless communications via cognitive dimension: An overview. *IEEE Network*, 25:50–56, March/April 2011, doi: 10.1109/MNET.2011.5730528.
[6] T. Chen, H. Zhang, Z. Zhao and X. Chen. Towards green wireless access networks. In *Proceedings of ChinaCom 2010*, Beijing, August 2010.
[7] L. Pelusi, A. Passarella and M. Conti. ONing: Data forwarding in disconnected mobile ad hoc networks. *IEEE Commun. Mag.*, 44(11), 2006.
[8] R. Thomas, D. Friend, L. DaSilva and A. McKenzie. Cognitive networks: Adaptation and learning to achieve end-to-end performance objectives. IEEE Commun. Mag., 44(12):51–57, December 2006.
[9] Phydyas Project, http://www.ict-phydyas.org/.
[10] Rocket Project, http://www.ict-rocket.eu/.
[11] Sendora Project, http://www.sendora.eu/.
[12] Winner Project, http://projects.celtic-initiative.org/winner+/.
[13] Crown Project, http://www.cs.qub.ac.uk/fp7-crown/.

[14] EUWB Project, http://www.euwb.eu/.

[15] ETSI TC RRS http://www.etsi.org/website/technologies/RRS.aspx.

[16] ETSI TR 102 682 v1.1.1, Reconfigurable Radio Systems (RRS); Functional Architecture (FA) for the Management and the Control of Reconfigurable Radio Systems, July 2009.

[17] ETSI TR 102.683, v1.1.1, Reconfigurable Radio Systems (RRS); Cognitive Pilot Channel (CPC), July 2009.

[18] S. Buljore, H. Harada, P. Houze, K. Tsagkaris, O. Holland, S. Filin, T. Farnham, K. Nolte and V. Ivanov. Architecture and enablers for optimised radio resource usage. *The IEEE P1900.4 Working Group Communications Magazine, IEEE*, 47(1):122–129, January 2009.

[19] ETSI, TR 102 838 V1.1.1 Reconfigurable Radio Systems (RRS); Summary of feasibility studies and potential standardization topics, 2009–2010.

[20] OneFIT Project, http://www.ict-onefit.eu/.

[21] UniverSelf Project, http://www.univerself-project.eu/.

[22] Cisco Visual Networking Index: Forecast and Methodology, http://www.cisco.com/en/US/solutions/collateral/ns341/ns525/ns537/ns705/ns827/white_paper_c11-481360.pdf.

[23] Global e-Sustainibility Initiative (GeSI). SMART 2020: Enabling the low carbon economy in the information age, http://www.theclimategroup.org/assets/resources/publications/Smart2020Report.pdf.

[24] Network Simulator 2 (NS-2). http://www.isi.edu/nsnam/ns/.

[25] ITU-T recommendation G.711. Aspects of digital transmission Systems.

[26] Charles E. Perkins. *Ad Hoc Networking*. Addision Wesley, 2001,

[27] T. Camp, J. Boleng and V. Davies. A survey of mobility models for ad hoc network research. *Wireless Communications & Mobile Computing (WCMC)*, Special issue on Mobile Ad Hoc Networking: Research, Trends and Applications, 2(5):483–502, 2002.

[28] N. Wang, K. Ho, G. Pavlou and M. Howarth. An overview of routing optimisation for IP traffic engineering. *IEEE Surveys and Tutorials*, 10(1):36–56, 2008.

[29] R. Teixeira, T. Griffin, A. Shaikh and G.M. Voelker. Network sensitivity to hot-potato disruptions. In *Proceedings ACM SIGCOMM*, August 2004.

[30] Awduche, D.O. MPLS and traffic engineering in IP networks. *IEEE Commun. Mag.*, 37(12):42–47, December 1999.

[31] B. Fortz, J. Rexford and M. Thorup. Traffic engineering with traditional IP routing protocols. *IEEE Commun. Mag.*, 40(10):118–124, October 2002.

[32] D.K. Goldenberg, L. Qiu, H. Xie, Y.R. Yang and Y. Zhang. Optimizing cost and performance for multihoming. In *Proceedings of ACM SIGCOMM 2004*, p. 79.

[33] A. Elwalid, C. Jin, S. Low and I. Widjaja. MATE: MPLS Adaptive Traffic Engineering. In *Proceedings IEEE INFOCOM*, pp. 1300–1309, 2001,

[34] M. Kodialam and T.V. Lakshman. Minimum interference routing of applications to MPLS traffic engineering. *IEEE INFOCOM*, pp. 884–893, 2000.

[35] M. Kodialam, T.V. Lakshman and S. Sengupta. Online multicast routing with bandwidth guarantees: A new approach using multicast network flow. *IEEE/ACM Trans. Networking*, 11(4):676–686, August 2003.

[36] K. Hinton, J. Baliga, M. Feng, R. Ayre and R.S. Tucker. Power consumption and energy efficiency in the internet. *IEEE Network Magazine*, Special issue on Energy-Efficient Networks, 25(2):6–12, March/April 2011.

[37] R. Bolla, R. Bruschi, A. Cianfrani and M. Listanti. Enabling backbone networks to sleep. *IEEE Network Magazine*, Special issue on Energy-Efficient Networks, 25(2):26–31, March/April 2011.

[38] A. Cianfrani, V. Eramo, M. Listanti, M. Marazza and E. Vittorini. An energy saving routing algorithm for a green OSPF protocol. In *Proceedings IEEE INFOCOM 2010*, San Diego (USA), 15–19 March 2010.

[39] S. Nedevschi, L. Popa, G. Iannaccone, S. Ratnasamy and D. Wetherall. Reducing network energy consumption via sleeping and rate-adaptation. In *Proceedings ACM, USENIX, NSDI*, 2008.

[40] S. Kandula, D. Katabi, S. Sinha and A. Berger. Flare: Responsive load balancing without packet reordering. *ACM Computer Communications Review*, 2007.

[41] D. Bertsekas and R. Gallager. *Data Networks*. Prentice-Hall, Englewood Cliffs, NJ, 1992.

[42] Rocketfuel: An ISP Topology Mapping Engine, http://www.cs.washington.edu/research/networking/rocketfuel/.

[43] B. Fortz and M. Thorup. Optimizing OSPF weights in a changing world. *IEEE JSAC*, 2002.

Biographies

Kostas Tsagkaris received his diploma (2000) and his PhD degree (2004) from the School of Electrical Engineering and Computer Science of the National Technical University of Athens (NTUA). He was awarded with the "Ericsson's awards of excellence in Telecommunications" for his PhD thesis. Since 2005 he is working as a senior research engineer and adjunct Lecturer in the undergraduate and postgraduate programs at the Department of Digital Systems of the University of Piraeus. He has been involved in many EU research projects including FP7/ICT UniverSelf, OneFIT and E3 and FP6/IST E2R I/II. His research interests are in the design, management and performance evaluation of wireless cognitive networks, self-organizing and autonomic networks, optimization algorithms, learning techniques and software engineering. He has published more than 100 papers in international journals and refereed conferences. He has also participated and contributed to EU and US standardization committees and working groups such as RRS and AFI-ISG groups in ETSI and IEEE DySPAN/P1900.4 group, where he has also served as Technical Editor of the published standard.

George Athanasiou received the diploma in Computer and Communications Engineering from University of Thessaly in 2005. He obtained his M.Sc. and Ph.D. degrees in Computer and Communications Engineering from the same University, in 2007 and 2010 respectively. Currently, he is a senior researcher at the laboratory of Telecommunication Networks and Services of the Digital Systems Department of the University of Piraeus working on the EU research project UniveSelf. From September 2005 to November 2010 he was a researcher at the Informatics and Telematics Institute (ITI) at the Center for Research and Technology Hellas (CERTH) working on several EU and National research projects: OPNEX, N-CRAVE, OneLab2, WIP, NEWCOMM, NEWCOM++, EuroNGI, EuroNF and CRUISE. From May 2009 to August 2009 he was an intern at Telefonica I+D, Internet Research Group, Barcelona, Spain, where he worked on the "ClubADSL: Bundling Wireless Connections" research project. The project has been recently awarded by Telefonica R&D as the best project of 2010 of all the R&D groups (including the centers in Barcelona, Madrid, Valladolid, Granada, Sao Paulo, Huesca, Mexico City) for its innovation. From August 2006 to November 2006 he was an intern at Polytechnic Institute of New York University. His research interests include the design and performance evaluation of wireless and fixed broadband networks, resource management, service and network management, cognitive networking, optimization techniques. He has authored numerous publications in these areas in international journals and refereed conferences. He is a member of the IEEE, ACM and the Technical Chamber.

Marios Logothetis received his Diploma and Master Degree from the Department of Digital Systems, University of Piraeus, in 2003 and 2006, respectively. Since January 2007 he is research engineer at the University of Piraeus, Laboratory of Telecommunication Networks and Services. He has been involved in several European projects (WinHPN, FP6/ IST E2rII and E3). At the moment he participates to the EU-funded FP7/ICT OneFIT (Opportunistic Networks and Cognitive Management Systems for Efficient Application Provision in the Future InterneT) project (7.2010-12.2012) and to the EU-funded FP7/ICT Univerself Integrated Project (2010-2013). Currently, he is a research engineer and PhD candidate at the University of Piraeus, Laboratory of Telecommunication Networks and Services. His main interests include management and performance evaluation of mobile ad hoc networks and wireless sensors, through simulations.

Yiouli Kritikou received her diploma in 2003 and her Ph.D. degree in 2009 from the Department of Digital Systems in University of Piraeus. Since September 2003 she is research engineer at the University of Piraeus, Laboratory of Telecommunication Networks and Services. As of January

2011, Dr. Kritikou conducts a post-doc research in Advanced Services in the context of the Future Internet. She has participated to the FP7/ ICT E3 (End-to-End Efficiency) Project (01.2008-12.2009), to the FP6/ IST Project E2R I/ II (01.2004-12.2007), as well as in a number of other national and international projects. Currently she is working in the FP7/ICT OneFIT (Opportunistic Networks and Cognitive Management Systems for Efficient Application Provision in the Future InterneT) Project (7.2010-12.2012), the FP7/ICT UniverSelf Integrated Project (09.2010-08.2013) and the FP7/ICT ACROPOLIS (Advanced Coexistence technologies for Radio Optimization in Licensed and unlicensed Spectrum) Network of Excellence (10.2010-09.2013). Her research interests are in the design, specification and development of services for wireless networks, concentrating on user profile, ubiquitous service delivery and technoeconomic aspects of services delivery.

Dimitrios Karvounas received his diploma from the School of Applied Mathematics and Physical Sciences of the National Technical University of Athens in 2007. He obtained an MSc in Digital Communications and Networks from the Department of Digital Systems of the University of Piraeus, Greece in 2009. Since February 2010 he is pursuing a PhD in Cognitive and Autonomous Management Techniques of the Future Internet and is a Research Engineer at the University of Piraeus Research Center (UPRC).

Panagiotis Demestichas, Associate Professor, received the Diploma and the Ph.D. degrees in Electrical and Computer Engineering from the National Technical University of Athens (NTUA). From December 2007 he is Associate Professor at the University of Piraeus, in the department of Digital Systems. Most of his current research activities focus on the Information Communication Technologies (ICT) Projects, partially funded by the European Commission under the 7th Framework Programme (FP7) for research and development. More specifically, he is the Project Coordinator of the ICT OneFIT (Opportunistic Networks and Cognitive Management Systems for Efficient Application Provision in the Future Internet) Project, he serves as the deputy leader of the Unified Management Framework workpackage in the ICT UniverSelf Project and as person in charge of administrative, scientific and technical/technological aspects in the ICT AC-ROPOLIS (Advanced coexistence technologies for Radio Optimisation in Licenced and Unlicensed Spectrum) project. Since January 2004 he has been the chairman of Working Group 6 (WG6) of WWRF, now titled "Cognitive Networks and Systems for a Wireless Future Internet" and he was the technical manager, from November 2008 until March 2010, of the "End-to-End Efficiency" (E3) project. His research interests include the design and performance evaluation of wireless and fixed broadband networks, software engineering, service and network management, algorithms and complexity theory, and queuing theory. He has several publications in these areas in international journals/ magazines and refereed conferences. He is a member of the IEEE, ACM and the Technical Chamber of Greece. He is the director of the M.Sc. program "Techno-economic Management and Security of Digital Systems", Department of Digital Systems, University of Piraeus, and he will be the head of the Department of Digital Systems, of the University of Piraeus, from September 2011 on.

The Use of Mobile Communication in Traffic Incident Management Process

S. Mandzuka,[1] Z. Kljaić[2] and P. Škorput[1]

[1]Department of Intelligent Transportation Systems, Faculty of Traffic Science, University of Zagreb, Vukelićeva 4, 10000 Zagreb, Croatia; e-mail: {sadko.mandzuka, pero.skorput}@fpz.hr; [2]Ericsson Nikola Tesla d.d., Krapinska 45, 10000 Zagreb, Croatia; e-mail: zdenko.kljaić@ericsson.hr

Received 25 June 2011; Accepted: 5 July 2011

Abstract

In cases of major traffic or other incidents it is very important to manage events dynamically in real time for one primary reason, i.e. in order to reduce death causalities and other technical and technological damages. A unique name for this system is Incident Management System. The critical point in the traffic incident management chain is the procedure after detecting the incident and the appropriate verification thereof. It is the process of informing other participants in road traffic. This paper gives a description of one such technology, known as Cell Broadcasting. A technological overview of the system along with its applications and experience in real-life environment is given here.

Keywords: intelligent transportation systems, Incident Management System, Cell Broadcasting, location based broadcasting.

1 Introduction

Everyday life in most cities of the world is becoming more dynamic. Growing needs of the population of urban areas are realized through continued

Journal of Green Engineering, 413–429.

increase in mobility and requirements for quality and travel safety. Urban and transportation planners are faced with many demands on the one hand and infrastructure constraints on the other hand. Increased mobility adversely affects the environment and the climate, human health, quality of life, social conditions and safety aspects of people and the wider society. We do not and cannot give up mobility, so we look for answers that introduce innovative, sustainable and energy efficient solutions that will contribute to the quality of life of citizens. Increased mobility has resulted in a significant increase in road traffic incidents and the induced damages and costs [1].

An "incident" is defined as any non-recurring event that causes a reduction of roadway capacity or an abnormal increase in demand. Such events include traffic crashes, disabled vehicles, spilled cargo, highway maintenance and reconstruction projects, and special non-emergency events (e.g., ball games, concerts, or any other event that significantly affects roadway operations). Although the problems most often associated with highway incidents consequence is traveler delay, by far the most serious problem is the risk of secondary crashes. Another related issue is the danger posed by incidents to response personnel serving the public at the scene.

Other secondary effects of incidents include:

- Increased response time by police, fire, and emergency medical services.
- Lost time and a reduction in productivity.
- Increased cost of goods and services.
- Increased fuel consumption.
- Reduced air quality and other adverse environmental impacts.
- Increased vehicle maintenance costs.
- Reduced quality of life.
- Negative public image of public agencies involved in incident management activities [2].

Road traffic incident management is a functional part of the holistic approach to solving traffic problems known under the term Intelligent Transportation System (ITS). The advanced development of communication and navigation technologies and their implementation in various phases of incident management can significantly reduce the consequences of incident event such as congestion, delay, pollution and especially dangerous secondary incidents [3].

Real-time incident management in traffic comprises coordination activities undertaken by several actors in order to reduce the negative impact, i.e., recovery of the traffic flow to the conditions of normal flow. One of the basic problems in incident management is the warning of other participants in traffic, as well as effective coordination of various organizations, i.e., services included in this process [4, 5]. Besides, incident management comprises also legal regulations which require careful planning of all segments. The success of the incident management lies in careful development of clear (and efficient) instructions and procedures, which are acceptable and understandable for all the involved services, organizations and individuals. One of the important conditions to achieve this is high-quality communications among the participants, i.e. information transparency and real-time data flow. Absence of such an approach which combines cooperation, communication and training, represent one of the main reasons of inefficient incident management process, today [6, 7].

The critical point in the traffic incident management chain is the procedure after detecting the incident and the appropriate verification thereof. It is the process of informing other participants in road traffic (special importance are the motorists) by using different technologies. Motorist information involves activating various means of disseminating incident-related information to affected motorists. Media used to disseminate motorist information include the following:

1. Commercial radio broadcasts.
2. Highway advisory radio (HAR).
3. Variable message signs (VMS).
4. Telephone information systems.
5. In-vehicle or personal data assistant information or route guidance systems.
6. Commercial and public television traffic reports.
7. Internet/on-line services.
8. A variety of dissemination mechanisms provided by information service providers.

Motorist information needs to be disseminated as soon as possible, and beyond the time it takes clear an incident. In fact, it should be disseminated until traffic flow is returned to normal conditions. This may take hours if an incident occurs during a peak period, and has regional impacts [2]. Recently, mobile (wireless) communications and their associated technologies and services have become increasingly important.

The development of wireless communications systems and their application in everyday life of citizens have enabled the use of mobile communications technology in urban processes, and opened the possibility of entirely new solutions that until now could not be realized. This new, technologically advanced solutions based on mobile communications systems have opened new possibilities in the creation of an urban and traffic policy, which should serve the increasing population needs to ensure their mobility, accessibility, efficiency, rationality of energy and environmental conservation.

The penetration of mobile communications is growing rapidly levels of 90% coverage are no longer exceptions [8]. Telecom operators, due to competition and saturation, are offering new services and focus on differentiation through value-added services.

This paper provides the description of one such technology, known as the Cell Broadcasting. In Section 2 a general model of Traffic Incident Management System is described. In particular, the importance of timely information about traffic incidents is pointed. The problem of traffic congestion caused by the incident is described. Some features of the Cell Broadcasting technology and some systemic functions are described in Section 3. The basic features of its architecture and a description of some specific interfaces are given. In Section 4, several examples of using Cell Broadcasting are shown. Some possibilities of GIS interfaces are presented. The concluding part gives the basic results of the work and the guidelines for future research.

2 Traffic Incident Management Process Model

There are several different events that influence the normal or desired traffic flow in road network. In [4] the following events are identified which may lead to temporary reduction in road network capacity (compared to requirement):

- vehicle-conditioned incidents, ranging from minor vehicle damage to multiple accidents with the injured and fatalities;
- debris/barriers on the road;
- maintenance activities;
- unpredicted congestions; and
- any combination thereof.

Another cause is extreme weather conditions, such as heavy rain or storms. Planned events (e.g., sport/cultural activities) or repeating events (e.g., peak congestions in the cities), are less interesting here due to the possibility of planned action.

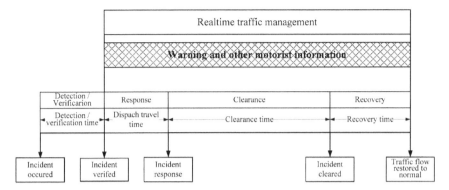

Figure 1 Phases in incident management.

The incident management process, as shown in Figure 1, is divided into four phases: incident detection and verification, incident response, clearance of the incident and recovery to normal traffic flow.

Incident detection may be defined as a process of identifying the space and time coordinates of the incident (incident situation) and possible nature of the incident itself. Incident detection methods are realized by private calls (phone, mobile phones), calls from SOS road phones, police report, report of the patrolling services and the operation of the automatic incident detection system. Incident verification means checking, which is used to determine the exact position and nature of the incident. In this way the possibility of responding to false alarms is reduced. Incident verification is carried out by the employees using the image obtained by specialized cameras (CCTV), or based on the comparison of several incoming calls about the incident.

The next step is very important. It is necessary to inform (warn) all participants in this road section about the nature of the incident. Implementation of this type of systems reduces the negative consequences of adverse events or sometimes an early warning of danger results in the adverse events not occurring. Figure 2 shows the relationship between the size of damage made in relation to the starting time of reaction. The figure is a display of statistically processed information on fires and their consequences. The diagram shows the impact of the shortest response of human and technical resources. It also shows the effect of sending real-time management information and alerts to people in danger, and in some cases, to participants in traffic approaching a site affected primarily or secondarily by consequences of accidental events [9, 10].

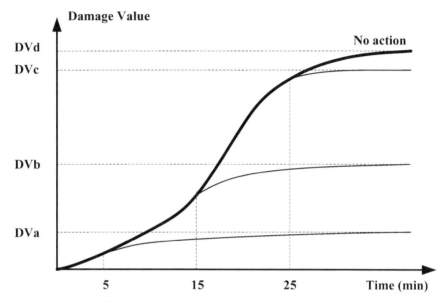

Figure 2 Quantity of caused damage in relation to initial response time.

We see from Figure 2 that if the intervention, which can range from intervention management of informing people to physical rescue of endangered, started after only 5 minutes, according to curve (a) the damage remained at the DVa level. If the intervention starts later, after 25 minutes, the damage was much higher, at DVd level.

Similarly, Figure 3 graphically shows the effect of reducing the cumulative arrivals of vehicles due to traffic flow diverting to alternative routes via cell broadcast messages about the emerged incidental situation [4, 11]. Also, as a positive consequence the response time of urgent services is shortened at the incident the situation due to the decrease (diversion) of traffic flow, and instructions to drivers on how to conduct themselves as they approach the place of incident.

Timely and accurate incident management and provision of information in real or near real time can significantly reduce the unwanted side effects that can exceed several times the incident that caused them.

According to the experience of leading projects in this area, it is generally considered that one minute lost for detection and verification requires four minutes to normalize the traffic flow.

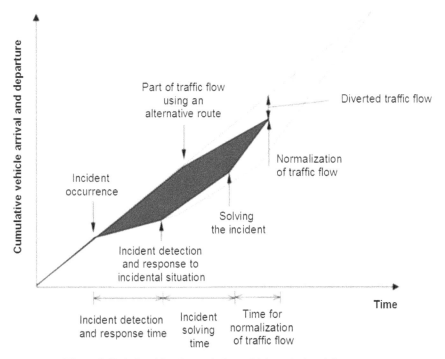

Figure 3 Relationship of cumulative vehicle arrival and departure.

3 Basic Technical Characteristics of Cell Broadcasting

The key to successful delivery of mobile services with added value is in finding the right combination of network services and content. An example of such a combination of content and functionality of the mobile network is providing the location-based technology, recently often used in entertainment and marketing industry.

These innovative telecom services began to develop more strongly after 2000. One of the services is "Location-qualified telecom messaging" which allows end users to receive different kinds of "push" specific information in relation to their current location, from multiple senders. One of the pioneering services in this area is the cellular broadcast system for sending telecom messages for emergency activities. Such services are based on sending alphanumeric messages to mobile phones (cell phones) that are found in a particular area that is dynamically determined by the content provider. The

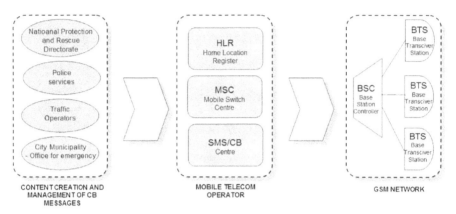

Figure 4 Functional diagram of cell broadcast system.

smallest area to which the content provider can send the contents is a radio cell, and the largest is a complete wireless network.

The Cell Broadcast System distributes information in a message format, very similar to the familiar SMS messages. These messages can be in a text or binary form. The length of a message is between 1 and 15 pages of 82 bytes (93 characters). A very important feature of this system is the distribution of information to a large number of users in a very short time. Processing required for the distribution of information is completely independent of the number of users that receive the information. The end user determines what information is to be presented to him and whether he wishes to receive this content. There are more than 65,000 channels available (in the ETSI terminology called "Message Identifiers"), each corresponding to a particular type of information.

The user individually activates and deactivates the reception of the first 999 broadcast channels. The rest of the channels must be activated via the OTA. Moreover, such a messaging system offers a range of unique functionalities such as support for sending specific information about location.

Apart from features provided by work in real time, the terminal required to receive broadcast information is continuously with the user, so he can read it immediately upon message delivery.

The system architecture of "location-qualified telecom messaging" gives the operator complete control over the network topology, whether it is a GSM or a UMTS (Universal Mobile Telecommunications System) network (Figure 4).

It also allows the content provider to work under largest load and with most complex cellular networks with their frequent changes. This is accomplished by dividing the system into two components, usually placed in two domains:

- Cell Broadcast Center (CBC) is a network element in the mobile network, which sends broadcast messages to a specific radio cells.
- One or more Cell Broadcast Entities (CBE) are connected to the CBC, and can be used locally (by operators) and remotely (by independent content providers) to define and send telecom messages with location importance.

Using the Cell Broadcast function, the end user selects relevant information, while blocking all other information. Received Cell Broadcast messages are displayed instantly on the display of the cell phone, or can be stored as Short Message Service (SMS) in the memory for later reading. The user selects relevant information by activating the so-called Cell Broadcast Channel (in ETSI terminology: "Message Identifiers").

This kind of telecom messaging supports messages in several languages, encoded in the ETSI Default Alphabet and Unicode (UCS2), as defined in [GSM 03.38 Phase 2+] and [3GPP TS 23.038] [12, 13].

Furthermore, such information can be sent in binary format for processing using machine-to-machine applications). A range of applications can take advantage of Cell Broadcast technologies, including the following examples:

- Traffic signs and information boards along the road can be equipped with mobile receivers.
- Dispatching systems can use the CB messages to send information to vehicles (taxis, police or firefighters).
- Traffic information for the navigation systems.

User interfaces of today's mobile phones support different procedures to activate the Cell Broadcast channel. Although manufacturers of mobile terminals develop and enhance functions, it is extremely important for the service of content providers to facilitate the activation of the Cell Broadcast channels. There are two ways to do this:

- Using the index message.
- Use the activation via Over the Air (OTA) – of services and tariff changes.

The index message is a specially formatted CB message with which channels from the menu can be selected and activated.

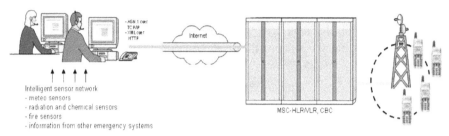

Figure 5 Cell broadcast system architecture.

In the case of activation via OTA, remote activation of CB channels (e.g., via a website) can be done by sending a binary SMS (also referred to as an OTA message) to the mobile device which updates the Subscriber Identity Module (SIM) card and activates the CB channels.

In addition to improving the user interface, activation of CB channels via OTA can provide a CB charging service (or its activation).

The center for location-specific telecom messaging is the central point for distribution of CB messages via a GSM network or a UMTS network. CBE submit broadcast claims to the CBC [14, 15]. Several CBE can be also interfaced to the center. CBC will address the appropriate cell controllers (Base Station Controller in a GSM network and Radio Network Controller in a UMTS network), which in turn will ensure the transmission of broadcast messages by the corresponding radio cells (Base Transceiver Station in a GSM Network and Node-B in a UMTS network). CBC supports a number of cell controllers in accordance with ETSI standards.

3.1 Interfaces for Cell Broadcast System

The CBE-CBC interface allows the CBE access to functions of the CBC. The interface accepts requests, processes them and transfers error messages or confirmation to the CBE. Message encoding (e.g., Universal Character Set 2) is transparent to the CBE-CBC interface.

The CBC provides two protocols for access to CBE:

- Protocol based on ASN.1.
- Protocol based on HTTP/XML.

CBE is connected to the CBC Center via LAN or a network interface, such as ISDN, X.25 or the Internet (Figure 5).

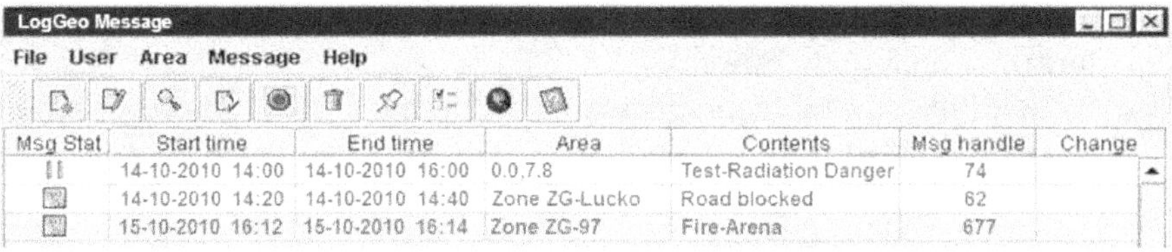

Msg Stat	Start time	End time	Area	Contents	Msg handle	Change
	14-10-2010 14:00	14-10-2010 16:00	0,0,7,8	Test-Radiation Danger	74	
	14-10-2010 14:20	14-10-2010 14:40	Zone ZG-Lucko	Road blocked	62	
	15-10-2010 16:12	15-10-2010 16:14	Zone ZG-97	Fire-Arena	677	

Figure 6 Alphanumeric cell broadcast system interface.

In the CBC, bandwidth control is performed on the CBE-CBC interface. That means when CBE exceeds the configured maximum bandwidth, the CBC will slow down sending replies.

Commands for cell controllers are provided with a list of cells, identifying the radio cells involved in commands. The cell controller is also responsible for the repetition of CB messages at a certain frequency. When a CB message is stopped, the cell controller reports the number of broadcasts by radio cell. ETSI has defined a standard for this interface (GSM 03.49 and [3GPP TS 25.419]), which the CBC supports. The CBC also supports interfaces to cell controllers that are not in accordance with ETSI standards.

The replies of the cell controller can change the internally maintained status variables of cell controllers and radio cells. The CBC attempts again to send failed messages for a configurable number of times. If after these attempts, the command is still not accepted, the command will be cancelled.

The CBC Center can be controlled remotely using the OMC (Operations and Maintenance Centre) via the web interface (Figure 6). Functions which the web interface provide are basic functions such as:

- start up and shut down of the CBC or its parts,
- entering basic information about the system (for e.g., position of a radio cell or which cell controller controls a specific radio cell),
- monitoring CBC activity.

The same functionality is provided in the CBC. An SNMP interface is available for remote monitoring of alarms.

The CBC automatically imports data on the topology of the GSM and the UMTS network (i.e. the relationship between radio cells and cell controllers) with file import tools. Data must be presented in the files, transferred using a file transfer protocol (FTP).

For a network element such as a Cell Broadcast Center, characteristics such as availability and capacity are of decisive importance.

Basic features are:

- Scalability, CBC can be implemented as CBS Smart (entry level platform), or dual-node Power CBS.
- Availability, several techniques are used in the CBC to improve system availability (Fail-take: if one node fails the other will take over.

3.2 Comparison of Cell Broadcast System and Short Message Service

SMS is one-to-one technology whereas CB is one-to-many. This significantly impacts the cost structure of such services allowing for easier network dimensioning. In an average network it would take 100 SMS with the same content approximately 30 seconds to reach its destination, whereas in a CB-enabled network, a similar message transmission takes 30 seconds to reach all end users tuned into a CB channel, up to several million at a time. Unlike SMS, the time to broadcast a message over a CB channel is insensitive to the number of subscribers scheduled to receive the message. In a typical CB, a message can be sent within 30 seconds to all handsets. Efficiency of communicating the message does not decline in peak hours and CB does not use the signaling network (IN7) to carry messages as with SMS. Some basic characteristics of Cell Broadcast System and Short Message Service are presented in Table 1.

4 Application of Cell Broadcasting in Traffic

The main application of Cell Broadcasting in traffic is sending alphanumeric messages for location-specific alarms and messaging within the framework of mobile telecommunications network. The main purpose is to warn and inform motorist and other participants about the event in this road section. Also, same system can be used to inform about other incidents such as natural disasters, infrastructure or chemical accidents, and terrorist or other security incidents. In Japan, since 2008, DoCoMo (Japan's premier mobile provider of leading-edge mobile voice, data and multimedia services) has implemented an alarm and messaging system for dangerous weather conditions and alert for earthquakes using the cell broadcast service. New York City in 2007 launched the "Crisis text via CB" project intended for early warning of citizens. The Indian operator BSNL (Broadband – Bharat Sanchar Nigam Ltd) has introduced a cellular broadcast of important information on disaster, as well as crisis management. The U.S. FEMA (Federal Emergency Management Agency) under the Department of Homeland Security in the United States implements

Table 1 Basic characteristics of SMS and CBS [16].

Characteristic	Short Message Service	Cell Broadcast Service
Handset compatibility	All handsets support SMS	Most handsets support CBS except Few numbers.
Transmission form	Unicast and Multicast communication	Broadcast service. Message received indiscriminately by every handset within broadcast range
Mobile number dependency	Dependent. Foreknowledge of mobile number(s) is essential	Independent. Message is received on activate broadcasting channel
Location dependency	Independent. User receives the message anywhere	Dependent. Targets one cell or more
Geo- information	Achieved by obtaining cell ID from the network operator	Cell(s) location is known for broadcaster beforehand
Service barring	No barring	Received only if the broadcast reception status is set to "ON"
Reception	Message is received once the mobile is switched on	No reception if handset is switched on after broadcasting
Congestion and delay	Affected by network congestions. Immense number of SMS may produce delays	Congestion is unlikely as CBS are sent on dedicated channels. Almost no delays except if received in poor coverage area
Delivery failure	Network overload might cause delivery failure	Busy mobile handset might fail to process a CBS message
Delivery confirmation	Sender can request delivery confirmation	No confirmation of delivery
Repetition rate	No repetition rate	Can be repeated periodically within 2 to 32 minutes intervals
Language format	Identical to all receivers	Multi-language messages can be broadcast on multiple channels simultaneously
Spamming	Some mobile service providers support internet connectivity. Internet-based SMS spamming is possible	Not possible expect through uncontrolled access to mobile network infrastructure and lack of safeguards by an irresponsible service provider

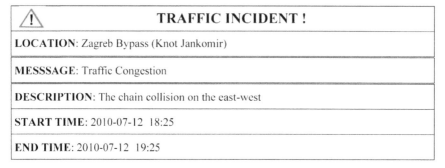

Figure 7 Example of traffic messaging [17].

the "Emergency Cell Broadcast Network" system for cities and areas till now frequently threatened by natural disaster.

Several operators and content providers develop traffic information services in real time. Two main types can be distinguished in these applications. One is the basic version in which location and traffic information is sent to users and displayed as text messages on their mobile devices. More advanced versions of these services are continually sending dynamic information on road conditions and their display on a navigation system (Figure 7).

For content providers, Cell Broadcast is a unique way of distributing information to large groups of users. Combining geographic information with demographic information, the content provider can target specific areas in a very advanced and effective manner. The areas are selected using the alphanumeric designation of the CBS or with Geographical Information System (GIS), and using an intuitive graphical user interface for entry of text messages and parameters (Figure 8).

Mobile networks are constantly expanding with new radio cells. The Cell Broadcast Center automatically retrieves updated information about the network topology in a preset time. Newly-added cells are now used for all current messages whose broadcast area overlaps with the new cells. This process is automatic and transparent to the content provider.

5 Conclusion

Reactions to incident events in real time reduce material damage and human casualties. Such properties have systems for early warning, that allow dislocation of people out of vulnerable locations. Especially an important role is played by these telecommunications systems in traffic that is very dynamic

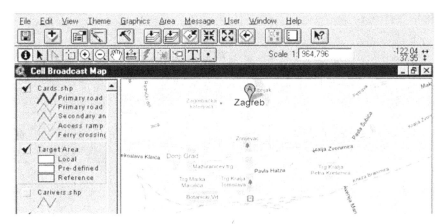

Figure 8 GIS interface for CBS.

and therefore complex in terms of management. The introduction of advanced telecommunications solutions increases safety in unfolding traffic reduces the number of casualties in traffic accidents and leads to faster response and actions by emergency services. Due to the success of implementation of such telecom systems, they become an integral part of the strategic program for design and deployment of regional ITS systems (ITS – Intelligent Transportation Systems). Tracking the number and severity of the consequences of accidents before and after the introduction of ITS provides a relatively objective quantification of the security gains and mitigates the effects of these events. Except in traffic incidents, similar processes and technology can be applied in the case of other emergencies, major accidents and disasters. Measuring the percentage reduction in response time is not a direct indicator of benefits, but is a very important factor. Reducing response time significantly affects the reduction of fatalities and prevent further casualties after the initial traffic (or other) accidents. Warning systems on highways improve driver perception of the accident scene and help reduce stress while traveling. Perception of safe travel is not only about reducing the number of accidents and their consequences, but also about increasing the perception of personal safety and security in transport. Also, dynamic and location-selective management of large incidents reduces the possibility of uncontrolled process (e.g., panic in humans). The introduction of new telecommunications technologies with the above properties, such as Cell Broadcast Systems, substantially increases the effectiveness of security systems in the public and the transport sector.

References

[1] S. Mandžuka, Z. Kljaić and P. Škorput. Application of ICT in the traffic incident management system. In *Proceedings CTI – MIPRO*, Vol. II, pp. 359–362, Opatija, 2011.

[2] Traffic Incident Management Handbook, Federal Highway Administration Office of Travel Management, November 2000.

[3] I. Bošnjak. *Intelligent Transportation Systems 1*, Faculty of Transport and Traffic Sciences, Zagreb, 2006 [in Croatian].

[4] P. Škorput. Real-time incident management system. M.Sc. Thesis, Faculty of Transport and Traffic Sciences, Zagreb, 2009 [in Croatian].

[5] P. Škorput, S. Mandžuka, N. Jelučić. Real-time detection of road traffic incidents. *Promet*, 22(4):273–283, 2010.

[6] C.L. Dudek, C.J. Messer and N.B. Nuckles. Incident detection on urban freeways. *Transportation Research Record*, 495:12–24, 1994.

[7] H. Dia, G. Rose and A. Snell. Comparative performance of freeway automated incident detection algorithms. In *Proceedings of Roads 96: Joint 18th ARRB Transp. Res. Conf. and Transit New Zealand Land Transp. Symp.*, pt. 7, pp. 359–374, 1996.

[8] Global mobile statistics 2011: All quality mobile marketing research, mobile Web stats, subscribers, ad revenue, usage, trends, ..., http://mobithinking.com/mobile-marketing-tools/latest-mobile-stats, visited June 2011.

[9] S. Mandžuka, Z. Kljaić and Z. Kordić. Mobile Telecommunication technology for Incident Management System. In *Proceedings of XVII Telecommunications Forum TELFOR*, 2009.

[10] Ch. Wattegama. ICT for Disaster Management, Asia-Pacific Development Information Programme, 2007.

[11] W.M. Evanco. The impact of rapid incident detection on freeway accident fatalities. Mitretek Center for Information Systems McLean, Virginia, 1996.

[12] Ericsson. Content Delivery System, FC 101 097/3, Stockholm, Sweden.

[13] Ericsson. Mobile Positioning System, FC 101 0351, Stockholm, Sweden.

[14] 3GPP TS 23.041; 3GPP TS 23.041. Technical realization of Cell Broadcast Service (CBS), 3GPP, V4.1.0

[15] GSM 03.41. Digital Cellular Telecommunications System (Phase 2+); Technical Realisation of the Short Message Service Cell Broadcast (SMSCB), ETSI.

[16] A. Aloudat, K. Michael and J. Yan. Location-based services in emergency management – From Government to citizens: Global case studies, Recent advances in security technology, Australian Homeland Security Research Centre, Melbourne, 2007, pp. 190–201.

Biographies

Sadko Mandzuka received his Univ. Ing. (1980), M.Sc. (1992), and Ph.D. (2003) degrees in Automatic Control from the Faculty of Electrical Engineering, University of Zagreb. He is currently Head of Transportation Telematics Chair, Faculty of Traffic Science, University of Zagreb. He has wide experience in the area of Floating Vessels Control Theory, Intelligent Transportation System, Artificial intelligence Technology, Traffic Incident Management System, etc. His main areas of interest are control problems in Intelligent Transportation Systems, applications of Artificial intelligence techniques to engineering optimization and Urban Traffic Incident Management System. He is author of more than 70 internationally reviewed publications. Professor Mandzuka received the prestigious Croatian State Award by the Ministry of Science in 1997. He is a founding member of the Croatian Robotic Association, Vice President of ITS-Croatia, and Collaborating Member of Croatian Academy of Engineering.

Zdenko Kljaić graduated in 1996 from the Faculty of Traffic and Transportation Engineering, University of Zagreb, and in 1997 received a Bachelor of Science in Electrical Engineering. He is currently attending the postgraduate masters study Information Management at the Faculty of Economics and Business, University of Zagreb. Furthermore, he studied in the field of strategic design and project management, and since 1998 has a specialization in designing and managing electrical construction projects in large and complex structures. He is a member of the Board of ITS Croatia (Intelligent Transport Systems), a member of the Assembly of Croatian Chamber of Traffic and Transportation Engineers. Since 2000, he has been permanently employed in Ericsson Nikola Tesla, Croatia, in the development of advanced solutions for Industry and Society.

Pero Škorput received his Dipl. Ing. degree (2002) and M.Sc. degree (2010) in the field of Transport and Traffic Science from University of Zagreb. He is currently postgraduate student in ITS. He has five years work experience in Ericsson Nikola Tesla as expert for telecommunication and System development. He is currently an Assistant at Faculty of Transport and Traffic Sciences for Courses: Basic of Traffic Engineering, Intelligent Transport System and Artificial Engineering. He is general secretary of Intelligent Transport Systems Croatia. His main research interests include Traffic Incident Management and Ontology Engineering in Transport and Traffic Domains.

A Heterogeneous Network for Energy Metering and Control

Enrico Paolini[1], Andrea Giorgetti[1], Simone Minardi[2] and
Marco Chiani[1]

[1]*DEIS/WiLAB, University of Bologna, Via Venezia 52, 47521 Cesena (FC), Italy*
e-mail: {e.paolini, andrea.giorgetti, marco.chiani}@unibo.it
[2]*I.co. Srl, Rimini (RN), Italy; e-mail: simone.minardi@icoworld.com*

Received 1 July 2011; Accepted: 7 July 2011

Abstract

We describe a heterogeneous network composed by wireless links and a power line communication (PLC) infrastructure, using the public lighting system. The network allows to measure consumption of gas, energy, water, etc., in an urban scenario with a large number of nodes, and to remotely control the lighting system for efficient energy usage. For the specific scenario where the network topology is known a priori, we describe a tool for network planning based on the simulation of the power line channel. Moreover, to improve PLC link throughput and reliability we analyze the possiblity to use multiple conductors to enable multiple input multiple output (MIMO) techniques. Finally, we describe a successfully implemented testbed for the proposed network.

Keywords: automatic meter reading, energy savings, heterogeneous networks, powerline communications, remote control.

1 Introduction

Power line communication (PLC) is a well-established technology for the telemanagement of outdoor lighting plants [1, 2]. There already are com-

Journal of Green Engineering, 431–445.

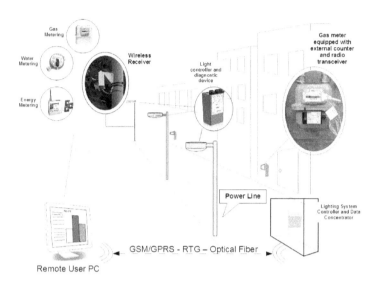

Figure 1 Reference scenario for a heterogeneous network based on the outdoor lighting system for smart AMR and control.

mercially available solutions for designing and manufacturing smart systems based on data communication over the main electricity (power line carriers), dedicated to the telemanagement of outdoor lighting plants and of both public and private building lighting systems. These solutions, devoted to energy saving, environment protection and improvement of life quality, are mainly based on low data rate PLC technologies.

In this paper we describe how the remotely controlled outdoor lighting system can be exploited to provide a low-cost, pervasive and heterogeneous wide area network for automatic meter reading (AMR) and control. AMR allows to automatically collect consumption, diagnostic, and status data from water, gas, electricity, or energy metering devices and to transfer these data to a central database for billing, troubleshooting, and analysis. A picture illustrating the basic system is reported in Figure 1.

The proposed system uses the outdoor lighting system as an infrastructure, putting a node on each lamp. Each node is connected by PLC to the backbone network, and contains a wireless transceiver (for instance, ZigBee, etc.) to reach customer energy metering devices. For lamps for which the PLC connection is not possible with the required quality of service (QoS), a wireless connection to the backbone network is used. In this respect, wireless and PLC technologies complement each other, depending on the capacities offered by the respective channels, disturbances, interference, and network topology.

The advantages of this solutions may be summarized as follows:

- *Wide coverage.* The lighting systems is already deployed worldwide so that, without additional infrastructure, a wide area system can be implemented.
- *Pervasivity.* The lighting systems is widespread and the lamps are very close to customers' metering equipments, so that the radio link can be made reliable with low energy consumption. In fact, the wireless node on the metering device must be battery equipped, and its consumption is directly related to the battery lifetime. Moreover, since lamps are quite ubiquitous and spatially close, in case of node failure the redundancy from nearby lamps can be exploited.
- *Power supply.* The electrical power needed for the wireless node is already available at each lamp, so no additional cabling is required, once the PLC/wireless node is placed on the lamp.

PLC communications can be divided in two categories: narrowband PLC (NB-PLC) and broadband PLC (BB-PLC). NB-PLC operates in the 3–500 kHz band and is characterized by low data rates, ranging from a few kbps to hundreds of kbps. For example, the *G3-PLC* standard for smart grid applications operates in the 35–91 kHz band and guarantees a data rate up to 33.4 kbps. BB-PLC operates in the 1.8–250 MHz band and can guarantee higher data rate links. Some of the standards that belongs to this category are *Home Plug 1.0*, *Home Plug AV*, *ITU-T G.hn* and *IEEE P1901*. For example, *Home Plug 1.0* can reach up to 14 Mbps while *Home Plug AV* data rate can be 200 Mbps [3].

The main challenge for the proposed system is represented by the design and implementation of a network with a large number of lamps equipped with a wireless interface, capable to offer smart metering functionalities in an area as large as possible. Note that the network performance is heavily affected by its topology. Therefore, a major design issue consists of the realization of a flexible *plug & play* network to keep the implementation simple and as independent as possible of the topology of the power lines to guarantee transparency to the users. Another crucial design issue is represented by network robustness to node outages, capable to by-pass wireless nodes experiencing an outage condition, dynamically overcoming the deterioration of the transmission channel. The network also requires multi-hop communic-

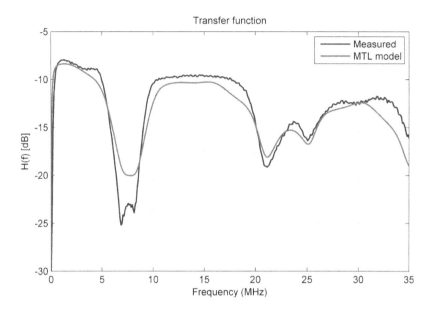

Figure 2 Example of measured channel frequency response. The channel frequency response predicted by the MTL model proposed in [6], compared with the frequency response measured through the pseudo-noise sequence generator.

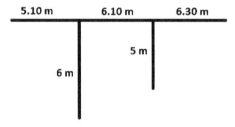

Figure 3 Topology of the network whose channel frequency response is depicted in Figure 2.

ation protocols and channel (e.g., frequency) reuse to cover wide areas. In summary, we target a *self-configurable* network with *cognitive* PLC/wireless nodes.

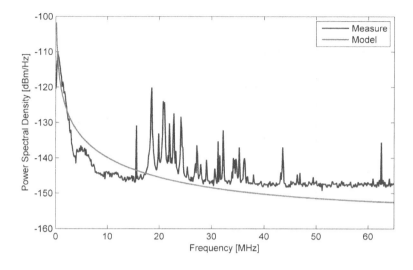

Figure 4 PLC noise measurement for an active network compared with the model for the background noise proposed in [7].

2 Software Tools to Predict the PLC Channel Impairments and Capacity

Within the context of the proposed system, PLC channel measurements have been performed for bandwidths of at least 30 MHz. For general references about channel models and measurements see [4–6]. The experimental setup comprises a pseudo-noise sequence generator with a chip rate of at least 100 Mchip/s, an analog to digital converter capable to export samples to a personal computer equipped with the software necessary for post-processing, and two couplers allowing to interface the instruments with a 220 V, 50 Hz power line. An example of measured channel frequency response is shown in Figure 2 for a network with two open branches whose topology is depicted in Figure 3, where it is evident the presence of notches in the transfer function. The performed measurement are in accordance with multipath models for power line signal propagation proposed in the literature (e.g. [4–6]). An extensive channel measurements campaign is currently taking place for the particular application scenario.

In addition to PLC channel frequency response measurements, we performed several measurements of the noise affecting the power line. An example for an active network is depicted in Figure 4, where the measured background noise is compared to the model proposed in [7]:

$$N(f) = \frac{1}{f^2} + 10^{-15.5} \text{ [mW/Hz].} \tag{1}$$

We observe a very good match between this model and the measurement at low frequencies. Moreover, we can observe the presence of narrow-band noise in the 15–40 MHz band, due to the interference of radio systems operating in this band and to several switches in the network being turned on and off.

3 Analysis of MIMO PLC Systems

In current PLC systems, the signal is transmitted and received exploiting the phase (P) and the neutral (N) conductors, leading to a single input single output (SISO) communication system. These systems are targeted to reach data rates as high as 200 Mbps over the $[1 \div 30]$ MHz frequency band. Their capacity may be calculated exploiting the simple formula

$$C_{\text{SISO}} = \sum_{n=1}^{N} \Delta_f \log_2 \left(1 + \frac{P_T\left(f_n\right) |H\left(f_n\right)|^2}{N_R\left(f_n\right)} \right) \text{ [bit/s]} \tag{2}$$

where N is the number of subcarriers exploited by the system (each subcarrier being associated with a band Δ_f), $N_R(f_n)$ is the power spectral density (PSD) experienced by the n-th subchannel (and assumed constant over each frequency interval of bandwdth Δ_f), and $H(f)$ is the transfer function that is obtained either by direct measurements or by applying, for instance, the MTL model [6]. For example, in the case of the background noise, $N_R(f)$ is given by the relationship (1). Note that the transmit PSD $P_T(f)$ yielding capacity is the outcome of a constrained optimization process based on the *water-filling* technique (see for example [9, chapter 10]), where the constraints are represented by the total transmitted power and by the PSD masks, currently imposing $P_T(f) < -30$ dBm/Hz for f up to 30 MHz and $P_T(f) < -50$ dBm/Hz otherwise.

In European and American power delivery networks, the number of available conductors is usually larger than two. In fact, at least a third conductor, namely the protective earth (PE) conductor, is available. It is therefore natural to try to exploit the three available conductors in order to obtain a MIMO system leading to higher capacities and data rates for the same transmitted power

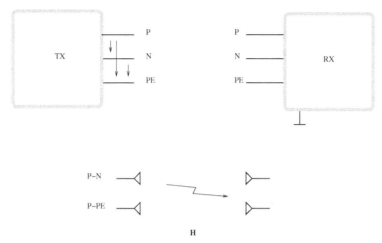

Figure 5 Ports illustration for a generic PLC network and analogy with a wireless MIMO system.

and bandwidth allocation. In wireless communication systems, MIMO consists of employing several antennas on both the transmitting and the receiving sides. In analogy with the wireless scenario, a MIMO PLC system exploits several conductors to achieve a diversity gain. Note that the role of a single antenna in MIMO wireless systems is now played by a pair of conductors. A generic MIMO PLC system exploiting the P, N, and PE conductors is depicted in Figure 5, where its analogy with a wireless MIMO system is emphasized.

Next, we discuss how the capacity of a MIMO PLC system can be estimated. With reference to Figure 5, three pairs of conductors are available for transmission, namely:

- *P (Phase)* and *N (Neutral)*;
- *PE (Protective Earth)* and *P (Phase)*;
- *N (Neutral)* and *PE (Protective Earth)*.

Because of the Kirchhoff law, only two of these three pairs can be exploited on the transmitter side, while in principle they can all be exploited on the receiver side (a fourth pair could be exploited as well by considering also the *common mode*). Letting n_T and n_R denote the number of ports on the transmitter and receiver sides, repectively, the channel matrix is given by

$$\mathbf{H}(f) = \begin{pmatrix} h_{11}(f) & \cdots & h_{1n_T}(f) \\ \vdots & \ddots & \vdots \\ h_{n_R 1}(f) & \cdots & h_{n_R n_T}(f) \end{pmatrix}$$

where the generic term $h_{nm}(f)$ represents the transfer function of the channel, relevant to the m-th input and n-th output ports.

By applying singular value decomposition (SVD) to the matrix $\mathbf{H}(f)$, it is possible to represent the MIMO system as a number of independent SISO channels, whose number equals the rank of $\mathbf{H}(f)$. Performing SVD, we obtain

$$\mathbf{H}(f) = \mathbf{U}(f)\mathbf{D}(f)\mathbf{V}^H(f),$$

where

- $\mathbf{U}(f)$ is an $n_R \times n_R$ unitary matrix, whose columns are the eigenvectors of $\mathbf{H}(f)\mathbf{H}^H(f)$;
- $\mathbf{D}(f)$ is an $n_R \times n_T$ diagonal matrix whose nonzero elements, $\sqrt{\lambda_j(f)}$, are the singular values of $\mathbf{H}(f)$;
- $\mathbf{V}^H(f)$ is the Hermitian transpose of the $n_T \times n_T$ matrix $\mathbf{V}(f)$, whose columns are the eigenvectors of $\mathbf{H}^H(f)\mathbf{H}(f)$.

SVD allows us to express the overall MIMO capacity as the sum of the capacities of the independent SISO systems. We then obtain the following expression for the capacity in bit/s:

$$C_{\text{MIMO}} = \frac{B}{N} \sum_{n=1}^{N} \sum_{j=1}^{\text{rank}(\mathbf{H})} \log_2 \left(1 + \frac{P_T(f_n)\lambda_j(f_n)}{N_R(f_n)} \right) \qquad (3)$$

where again the transmitted PSD is the outcome of an optimization process analogous to that described for the SISO case. In order to estimate the MIMO capacity, the entries of $\mathbf{H}(f)$ can be estimated using, for instance, the technique described in Section 2. An example of such measurements (conducted on a passive network) is depicted in Figure 6 for a (2×2) system based on the P-PE and P-N pairs of conductors, whose channel matrix is in the form

$$\mathbf{H}(f) = \begin{pmatrix} h_{11}(f) & h_{12}(f) \\ h_{21}(f) & h_{22}(f) \end{pmatrix}.$$

Note that $h_{12} \simeq h_{21}$ as expected.

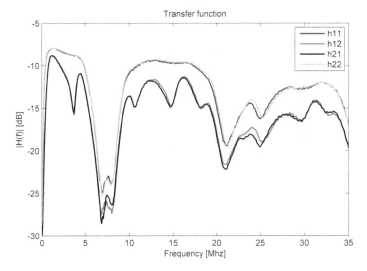

Figure 6 Measured entries of the **H**(f) matrix for a (2 × 2) MIMO PLC channel (passive network with two branches).

4 An Experimental Testbed for Energy Metering Through Heterogeneous Wireless/PLC Networks

The goal of the testbed is to implement a system remotely managing a public lighting infrastructure and, using the power line as communication medium to send and receive data, realize a network of sensors able to monitor methane gas consumption of surrounding homes (see Figure 7).

The system developed for this experimental testbed consists of an architecture divided into three levels: the spot light level, the street cabinet level and the server level. In each of these levels there is a device capable to perform different tasks. In particular, in the spot light a device is inserted called CADE (Control And Diagnostic Device), to control the on/off light switch, or to reduce the light intensity and carry out a diagnosis of the lamps and lighting devices (e.g., lamp starter, power factor correction capacitor). Each CADE uses the same power line to supply lighting when prompted and to communicate with devices in the street cabinet level, through NB-PLC. The main device in the street cabinet is a dedicated programmable logic controller, whose primary task is to manage up to 1024 CADE, send them commands for on/off light scheduling or reducing the brightness of each lamp, and to receive data from CADE about the status of each light circuitry. At the same

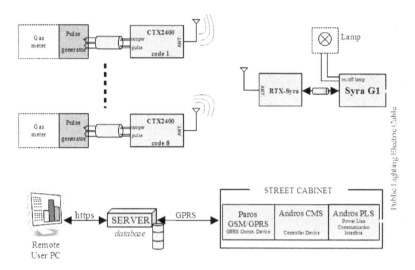

Figure 7 Testbed for outdoor-lighting-system-based heterogeneous network for smart energy metering and control.

time, using the GSM mobile network (or other network infrastructures based on, e.g., optical fiber), the controller communicates with the server manager, which is the last architecture level.

Through this architecture is then possible to deploy, on every pole of the public lighting infrastructure, a CADE for lamps management and diagnosis. Integrating the system, in particular the CADE, by device interface with radio communication capabilities, the system is able to communicate with hetero-geneous wireless devices, such as wireless sensor networks, with different radio technologies.

In the testbed we employed some CADE devices with a radio interface based on energy-efficient technologies that can operate in the 2.4 GHz ISM band. The heart of this interface is a common system-on-chip tailored for IEEE 802.15.4, and ZigBee smart energy applications. Thanks to this integration, the CADE device can act as a gateway node (CADE-G) for a wireless sensor network. For this experiment we used an ultra-low power wireless node to read the gas meters of homes located in the proximity of the public lighting infrastructure. Each network node, called the CTX2400, is connected to its gas meter diaphragm through a low-frequency pulse generator.

Each pulse induced by the gas meter corresponds to a certain volume (usually 1 dm^3/pulse) of consumed gas and reading by CTX2400 is performed continuously; to avoid manipulation, the CTX2400 monitors the integrity of the cable connection with the pulse generator through tamper, built-in sensor. Every hour, the CTX2400 sends to its gateway a radio packet containing the total detected consumption, the status of the tamper and the voltage level of its battery. The CTX2400 is compatible with the standard IEEE 802.15.4, thereby ensuring interoperability with other systems adopting the same standard, while the MAC layer and the application layer have been designed to ensure access to the channel using TDMA technique and a very low duty-cycle, in order to minimize battery consumption.

In particular, the CTX2400 has the following features:

- *Protocol Stack*. IEEE 802.15.4 compliant.
- *Power Consumption*. Ultra low sleep current equal to $0.4\,\mu$A and average current equal to $25.4\,\mu$A with a very low duty-cycle of 0.08% with 1 transmission per hour.
- *Battery Liftime*. Low cost lithium battery, totally integrated in the device. Lifetime of up to 7 years with 1 transmission per hour and up to 20 years with 1 transmission every 6 hour.[1]
- *Output power*. $+3.5$ dBm EIRP and up to 400 m coverage in line-of-sight scenario with point to point communication.
- *Security*. Data encryption with AES 128 bit to ensure secure data transmission.

The system has been running for six months and is monitoring the consumption of 115 households using 115 CTX2400 devices and 15 G-CADE devices; actually, CADE-G gateway is able to manage the communication with up to 8 CTX2400. The light spots controlled by the system are beyond 1500, while the involved street cabinets are 28. The entire system is managed through the use of a dedicated server, equipped with Linux operating system, through the use of web-based application which can be used to set the on/off/reduction scheduling of each single lamp as well as receive data about consumption of methane gas and make simple historical reports; it is also possible to keep under control the status of the wireless sensors network by viewing the status of the CTX2400 battery and tamper protection of the pulse generator.

The system has provided significant advantages, namely:

---

[1] This is a theoretical estimation that does not consider battery degradation.

- 35% reduction in consumption of public lighting, through control of the brightness of each lamp and removing anomalies such as undesired switch-on before sunset.
- 65% reduction on the maintenance costs of public lighting, monitoring possible failures at each light circuitry.
- Timely identification of possible leaks and failures in the gas distribution system by hourly monitoring of consumption.
- Billing consumption of gas methane based on real data and not on estimates, eliminating the need for periodic readings directly on each gas meter.

The experiment includes further developments on the system in the upcoming months, with the goal of enabling the sending of data and commands to the sensors network through the web browser. Another goal is to significantly increase the number of devices managed by each gateway and implement communications networks more complex than the simple star network in use, in order to increase the radio coverage of the system. In addition, several location-based services are already provided through the tastbed, such as access control in the town centre (through electromechanical bar control). Additional services could be implemented with minimal effort.

5 Conclusion

We described a heterogeneous network composed by wireless links and a power line communication system, using the public lighting infrastructure. For the specific scenario where the network topology is often known a priori, we presented a tool for network planning based on the simulation of the power line channel, with the possibility to use multiple conductors to enable MIMO techniques to improve PLC link throughput and reliability. Finally, we described a testbed of the network that allow measuring energy consumption, in an urban scenario with a large number of nodes, and to remotely control the lighting system for optimal energy usage.

References

[1] K. Dostert, *Powerline Communications*. Prentice-Hall, 2001.
[2] S. Galli and O. Logvinov. Recent developments in the standardization of power line communications within the IEEE. *IEEE Commun. Magazine*, 46(7):64–71, July 2008.
[3] S. Galli, A. Scaglione and Z. Wang. For the grid and through the grid: The role of power line communications in the smart grid. *Proc. IEEE*, 99(6):998–1027, June 2011.

[4] M. Zimmermann and K. Dostert. A multipath model for the powerline channel. *IEEE Trans. Commun.*, 50(4):553–559, April 2002.

[5] T.C. Banwell and S. Galli. A novel approach to the modeling of the indoor power line channel – Part I: Circuit analysis and companion model. *IEEE Trans. Power Delivery*, 20(2):655–663, April 2005.

[6] T.C. Banwell and S. Galli. A novel approach to the modeling of the indoor power line channel – Part II: Transfer function and its properties. *IEEE Trans. Power Delivery*, 20(3):1869–1878, July 2005.

[7] D. Benyoucef. A new statistical model of the noise power density spectrum for power-line communication. In *Proceedings of IEEE International Symposium on Power Line Commun. and Its App.*, Kyoto, Japan, 2003.

[8] C.L. Giovaneli, P.G. Farrell and B. Honary. Improved space-time coding applications for power line channels. In *Proceedings of IEEE International Symposium on Power Line Commun. and Its App.*, pp. 50–55, March 2003.

[9] T.M. Cover and J.A. Thomas. *Elements of Information Theory*. Wiley, 1991.

Biographies

Enrico Paolini received his Dr. Ing. degree (with honors) in telecommunications engineering and his Ph.D. degree in telecommunications engineering from the University of Bologna, Italy, in 2003 and 2007, respectively. While working toward the Ph.D. degree, he was Visiting Research Scholar with the University of Hawaii at Manoa. From 2007 to 2010, he held a postdoctoral position with the Department of Electronics, Computer Science and Systems (DEIS), University of Bologna, where he is currently Assistant Professor. His research interests include error-control coding (with emphasis on LDPC codes and their generalizations, iterative decoding algorithms, reduced-complexity maximum likelihood decoding for erasure channels), and radar sensor networks based on ultrawideband technology. In the field of error correcting codes, has been involved since 2004 in several activities with the European Space Agency (ESA). Dr. Paolini served on the Technical Program Committee at several IEEE International Conferences, and on the Organizing Committee of ICUWB 2011.

Andrea Giorgetti received his Dr. Ing. degree (magna cum laude) in electronic engineering and his Ph.D. degree in electronic engineering and computer science from the University of Bologna, Bologna, Italy, in 1999 and 2003, respectively. Since 2003, he has been with the Istituto di Elettronica e di Ingegneria dell'Informazione e delle Telecomunicazioni (IEIIT-BO) research unit at Bologna, National Research Council (CNR), Bologna. In 2005, he was a Researcher with the National Research Council.

Since 2006, he is Assistant Professor at the Second Faculty of Engineering at the University of Bologna, and he joined the Department of Electronics, Computer Sciences and Systems. During the spring of 2006, he was a Research Affiliate with the Laboratory for Information and Decision Systems, Massachusetts Institute of Technology, Cambridge, working on coexistence issues between ultra-wideband (UWB) and narrowband wireless systems. His research interests include ultrawide bandwidth communication systems, wireless sensor networks, and multiple-antenna systems. Dr. Giorgetti was TPC Co-Chair of the Wireless Networking Symposium, IEEE International Conference on Communications (ICC 2008), Beijing, China, May 2008; and TPC Co-Chair of the MAC track of the IEEE Wireless Communications and Networking Conference (WCNC 2009), Budapest, Hungary, April 2009.

Simone Minardi received his B.Sc. degree in telecommunications engineering and his M.Sc. degree (Laurea Specialistica) in electronics and telecommunications engineering both from the University of Bologna, Italy, in 2006 and 2009, respectively. Since 2009, he is system engineer and project manager at I.Co. s.r.l., working on the design and implementation of wireless networks for smart environments and wireless sensor networks for landslide monitoring and automatic meter reading.

Marco Chiani was born in Rimini, Italy, in April 1964. He received his Dr. Ing. degree (magna cum laude) in electronic engineering and his Ph.D. degree in electronic and computer science from the University of Bologna, Italy, in 1989 and 1993, respectively. He is a Full Professor of Telecommunications and the current Director of the Industrial Research Center on ICT, University of Bologna. During summer 2001, he was a Visiting Scientist with AT&T Research Laboratories, Middletown, NJ. He is a frequent visitor at the Massachusetts Institute of Technology (MIT), Cambridge, where he presently holds a Research Affiliate appointment. He is leading the research unit of the University of Bologna on cognitive radio and UWB (European project EUWB), on Joint Source and Channel Coding for wireless video (European projects Phoenix-FP6 and Optimix-FP7), and is a consultant to the European Space Agency (ESA-ESOC) for the design and evaluation of error correcting codes based on LDPCC for space CCSDS applications. His research interests include wireless communication systems, MIMO systems, wireless multimedia, low-density parity-check codes (LDPCC) and UWB. He is the past Chair (2002–2004) of the Radio Communications Committee of the IEEE

Communication Society and past Editor of *Wireless Communication* (2000–2007) for the IEEE Transactions on Communications. He is a Fellow of the IEEE.

Energy Consumption of Personal Computing Including Portable Communication Devices

Pavel Somavat[1] and Vinod Namboodiri[2]

[1]CCS Haryana Agricultural University, Hisar, Haryana, India
[2]Department of Electrical Engineering and Computer Science, Wichita State University, Wichita, KS 26260, USA; e-mail: vinod.namboodiri@wichita.edu

Received: 24 May 2011; Accepted: 19 July 2011

Abstract

In light of the increased awareness of global energy consumption, questions are being asked about the energy contribution of computing equipment. Although studies have documented the share of energy consumption by this type of equipment over the years, research has rarely characterized the increasing share contributed by the rapidly growing segment of portable, pervasive computing devices. Portable computing is widely predicted to be a dominant mode of computing and communication in the future, and accounting for its energy consumption is necessary to develop efficient practices. This work takes a fresh and updated look at energy consumption as the result of computing devices with regard to global consumption, and pays special attention to the contribution of portable computing devices. We further quantify the impact of energy consumed by the computing sector on the environment, and the cost of electricity for an average residential consumer. Finally, based on the results of this study, we provide recommendations for the computer networking community for sustainable portable/mobile computing.

Keywords: energy, electricity, computing, portable devices, environment, networking.

Journal of Green Engineering, 447–475.

1 Introduction

The increasing role of the Internet in our lives has ushered in a tremendous growth in computing devices governed by patterns such as the famous *Moore's Law*, which describes a long-term trend in the history of computing hardware that has continued for more than half a century, whereby the number of transistors that can be placed inexpensively on an integrated circuit has doubled approximately every two years. Computing devices are playing different roles in server farms, data centers, and office equipment, among others. There is increased awareness, however, in how the world consumes energy and its impact on the planet. Thus, it is natural to think about the impact of computing on the global energy consumption as well. There have been many studies that document this impact [1–3].

The world, however, is changing the way it accesses the Internet, and computing in general. The relevance of portable, battery-operated devices to handle computing and communication tasks is increasing. The first phone call over a GSM cellular phone occurred in 1991. By the end of 2007, half the world's population possessed such phones. This phenomenon is similar to the growth of computing devices in general, where central processing unit (CPU) processing power and capacity of mass storage devices doubles every 18 months. Such growth in both processing and storage capabilities fuels the production of ever more powerful portable devices. Devices with greater capabilities work with more data and subsequently have greater capability to communicate data. This has resulted in a similar exponential growth of wireless communication data rates as well the need to provide adequate quality of service.

There have been no studies to date that fully document the impact of the rapidly growing segment of portable computing devices on global energy consumption and what we can expect in the future. Such a study requires a detailed analysis of energy consumption by these devices as compared to computing devices in general, as well as an understanding of the magnitude of these numbers in terms of global energy consumption. This accounting also needs to include the impact not only in terms of energy, but also on the environment.

In this work, we profile the energy consumption of portable computing devices and account for their impact on global energy consumption. Our contributions in this work are the following:

1. We account for global energy consumption due to all computing devices that include server farms/datacenters, office equipment, and desktops.

Our statistics indicate that computing consumes more than 6% of the global electricity consumption.

2. We characterize the power consumption of portable computing devices like laptops and mobile phones, and account for their share of global energy consumption. We find that the share of energy consumed due to portable devices is 14% of the overall personal computing segment.[1]

3. We put the energy consumption due to computing devices in perspective of global electricity consumption and consider their broader impact. Our accounting indicates that emissions due to computing annually are equivalent to that produced by 10 million vehicles on the road. From the perspective of residential electricity consumption of an average consumer, the share due to computing is 3% in the US. However, when a populous, developing country like India is considered, computing consumes about 8% of the total share, due to the lower electricity consumption per household compared to the US.

4. We make recommendations to deal with the issue of energy consumption by portable devices based on the results of this paper that portable devices consume non-negligible energy.

These contributions are significant and novel due to the fact that we provide adequate detail about how our energy numbers are calculated for various computing sectors, including the fast-growing portable device segment. We expect that our paper will encourage researchers to identify the impact of individual computing sectors in terms of energy and to work towards more energy-efficient pervasive computing in the future. Without such detailed accounting, the notion that computing is a significant consumer of energy will never emerge from the shadows of other energy-consumer segments like transportation, appliances, and lighting. A preliminary version of this work appeared in [60] that presented results of our accounting study; based on subsequent feedback, updated data available, and additional data analysis, most of the key results and their insights have been updated and presented in this work including the addition of energy consumed due to the Internet infrastructure.

This paper is organized as follows: In Section 2, we account for the energy consumption from various sectors. In Section 3, we profile the energy con-

---

[1] We define the "personal computing segment" to include devices used on the front-end by consumers like laptops, mobile phones, and desktops, and devices used on the back-end like server farms/data centers, the Internet, and mobile infrastructure. We do not include office equipment like printers, copiers, etc., and consumer electronics like TVs, DVDs, etc.

sumption of individual portable computing devices. In Section 4, we estimate the total number of portable devices used globally. Subsequently, using numbers from Sections 3 and 4, we calculate the total energy consumption due to portable computing in Section 5. Also in Section 5, we present energy consumption statistics for the personal computing segment in the context of overall global electricity consumption. In Section 6, we examine the environmental impact in terms of emissions due to the personal computing sector, and the cost to consumers from a residential consumer perspective. Based on the results of our analysis of energy consumption from multiple perspectives, in Section 7, we make specific recommendations for keeping portable device energy consumption in check and preparing for a future in which the energy consumption due to computing cannot be ignored. Finally, in Section 8, concluding remarks are made.

2 General ICT Accounting

In this section, we account for the energy consumed by devices that fall into the general class of information and computing technology (ICT). This section is intended to familiarize the reader with trends in energy consumption, significant events happening in the area, projected growth, and environmental impact. We will narrow our focus to specific energy consumption numbers in Section 4.

2.1 Data Center/Server Farm Energy Consumption and CO_2 Emissions

Data centers or server farms are fast becoming a considerable source of energy consumption. Some of the factors driving this increase include the increasing popularity of web-based applications, an ever increasing number of information-hungry Internet users, streaming video and audio, the popularity of Internet-based social networking, and a need to store considerable data to satisfy user demand. Many large companies like Google, Microsoft, Yahoo, Ebay, Amazon, etc., are investing very heavily in establishing newer server farms to provide support to their respective customer queries. The emerging concept of cloud computing is fueling this development even further. However, the rapid increase in data centers implies drawing more and more power from the grid in order for them to function. This not only includes power to run the servers but also the energy involved in heating, ventilating, air conditioning (HVAC), and lighting. A large data center may require many megawatts of electricity, enough to power thousands of homes. Although not all data center servers are power intensive, those like search engines consume a considerable amount of power. According to Google, every query consumes about 1 kilojoules (KJ) [4]. Because of these data farms, estimates put Google's annual electricity consumption figures at approximately 0.63 million megawatt hours (MWh) costing more than US $38 million [5].

With the increase in global computation needs, these farms are set to multiply, thus becoming a real cause of environmental concern. In 2006, servers and data centers accounted for an estimated 61 million MWh, or 1.5% of US electricity consumption, costing about $4.5 billion. It is projected that the power consumption by US server farms in 2011 will reach 100 million MWh, an increase of 12.7% that will require about ten new nuclear or coal-powered generation plants [6]. Therefore, these farms are becoming electricity guzzlers and a considerable source of carbon dioxide (CO_2) emissions. The total CO_2 emissions globally is close to about 30 billion tons [7, 48], where the server farms alone contribute 200 million tons of CO_2. According to the Environmental Protection Agency (EPA), data centers in the US alone produced 44.4 million tons of CO_2 in 2007, and continuing trends mean that these centers will release 80–100 million tons of CO_2 in 2011 [6].

Extensive studies by Koomey in 2008 [9] were carried out to calculate the overall energy consumption by data centers and to predict future trends. The approximate energy consumption in 2005 was 153 million MWh, and building on this study, Pickavet et al. [10] estimated this figure to be 254 million MWh in 2008. Based on these studies and projections based on growth trends, we can estimate the overall energy consumption due to data centers in 2010 to be 350 million MWh. However, if we deduct the amount of energy consumed indirectly for HVAC and others, which is about the same as energy consumed directly for computation operations according to [9], we can estimate the direct energy consumption to be 175 million MWh.

2.2 Office Equipment Energy Consumption and CO_2 Emissions

According to Department of Energy projections ranging from 2005 to 2015 and published in 2005, office equipment will be the fastest-growing commercial end use between 2003 and 2025 [11]. The potential for energy savings in offices through devices employing various energy efficient designs was identified in the early 90s. The Energy Star Program was initiated in 1992 by the US EPA as an effort to reduce the energy consumption and greenhouse gas emissions from power plants. In 1993, EPA extended that program to include computers, monitors, and printers. The initial motivation was to extend the energy saving features of laptops to desktops and printers. These measures became popular partly due to governmental regulation that all the microcomputers, monitors, and printers purchased by federal agencies be Energy Star compliant [12]. Begun as a voluntary labeling program designed to promote energy efficient design in computer related products, this movement has been extended to more than 40,000 components ranging from homes and buildings to lighting. Since its inception in 1992, Energy Star has grown from a program focusing on personal computers to a multinational program promoting over 30 products across commercial and residential markets, with thousands of program partners [13]. According to the annual savings report published in March 2009, it is estimated that the program resulted in more than $19 billion in total energy bill savings, and at the same time reduced green house gas emissions by more than 43 million tons [14].

Motivated by the success of this program, various studies have documented the energy consumed by office equipment, with recommendations given to bring this number down; this has resulted in new start-ups with green technologies in mind [15]. A detailed study done in 2006 found that although power management modes of office computing devices are saving energy, there is still a considerable amount of energy being wasted when these devices are inactive. This study recommended that PCs be connected to networks for more savings potential [2]. Taking this approach even further, a Japanese study explored potential savings by shortening the power management delay time for office devices like PCs, displays, copiers, and laser printers. Results showed that such device management can save as much as 3.5 million MWh per year, which is nearly equal to 2% of commercial electricity consumption in Japan [3]. Therefore, even though a considerable amount of work has been done in the area of energy savings for office devices, much more can still be achieved.

2.3 Growth in Personal Computing Devices

Personal computing devices globally, like server farms and office equipment, have increased rapidly over the years becoming another major consumer of electricity. Data provided by the Computer Industry Almanac, through its annual briefings since 1993, give very detailed information for the total number of computers in use around the globe. Beginning in 1975, the approximate number of computers in use in the world was 0.3 million, of which 0.2 million were in the US. In the next five years, this number rose to 4 million, showing

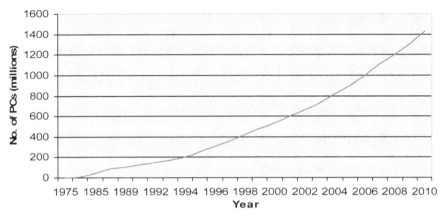

Figure 1 Our projected statistics for number of computers in use worldwide.

a 1233% increase. From 1980 to 1990, this increase was from 4 million to 116 million with a 2800% increase over the decade. The computer industry continued to grow at a remarkable pace in the 1990s, and the number of computers in use increased from 116 million in 1990 to 530 million in 2000, implying a 357% increase [16].

In the new millennium, this growth continued unabated, although the industry reached a relative state of maturity. Estimates by Forrester Research Institute forecast the total number of computers in 2015 to hit 2 billion, with countries like India, China, Brazil, and Russia accounting for more than 775 million new computers [17]. Similar estimates by Gartner expect this number to reach the 2 billion mark by 2014, forecasting the annual growth to be 12% per year [18].

Thus, from the above-mentioned statistics, the number of total computers in use can be estimated to be 1,300 million at the end of 2009 [16]. The increase in number of computers in use since 1975 and growth projections until 2010 are illustrated in Figure 1, based on [16, 17] which gives an estimate of 12% growth per year. Of the total number of computers in 2010 of 1,460 million, there are 1,000 million desktops and 460 million laptops, with the contribution of laptops increasing rapidly.

2.4 Other Related Work

Significant power is consumed by the mobile telecommunication infrastructure, including base stations. According to a study done by mobile communications giant Ericsson in 2007, communication infrastructure contributed to approximately 0.12% of global energy consumption and about 0.14% of global CO_2 emissions [19]. As an ever increasing number of people are becoming subscribers, this will further fuel the demand for extensive coverage networks, which in turn will draw more power from the grid. This will be especially significant in developing economies where current infrastructure is not enough to satisfy the increasing demand.

Rising awareness about the detrimental environmental effects of the increase in greenhouse gas emissions and increasing costs of energy has compelled a large number of companies and industrial segments to reconsider their priorities. Therefore, motivated by ethical or economical reasons, a large number of companies have started considering green practices. Huge savings attained by the Energy Star Program have also provided positive momentum in this direction, motivating companies like Nokia, Ericsson, Intel, Google, Microsoft, and others to go for innovation-ensuring energy-saving practices in their products. The concern for one industry has proved to be the bounty for others; in the UK alone, there are approximately 7,000 companies operating with environmental technologies, as the sector is set to grow to $34 billion by the end of the decade [15]. Increasing data-center energy costs and related emissions have put the entire industry in a spot of anxiety, and considerable effort is being made to ensure the most efficient practices. Countries like Iceland have started investing tremendously in data-center infrastructure to attract data centers, as most of the electricity is generated from clean sources, and also the cold weather in that part of the globe can be utilized for efficient cooling [20]. In addition to companies, academia is also playing its part by bringing these issues to the fore. Earlier in this section, we discussed a number of such studies concerning the documentation of results from the Energy Star implementation and similar other initiatives discussing various efficiency scenarios.

3 Portable Device Energy Profile

In this section we take a detailed look at the power consumption profile of the two common classes of portable devices: laptops and mobile phones. We believe these two classes to be representative of the spectrum of portable computing and communication devices. We obtain the power consumption profile of these devices through a combination of our own measurements and prior work by researchers. Our measurement was based on using the Kill-A-Watt meter [21]. This meter provides the instantaneous power consumption of any device plugged into it.

Table 1 Laptop power study.

Mode	Specification	Power consumptio when WNIC (W	Power consumption Idling with WNIC on	Power consumption when video streaming through WNIC (W)
HP pavilion dv4t	4GB RAM, 2GHz processor	30	31	32
Dell Inspiron	3GB RAM, 2GHz processor	21	24	36
Compaq Presario C30	2GB RAM, 2GHz processor	28	30	34
Dell Inspiron	4GB RAM, 2.2GHz processor	18	19	24
Aspire 4730Z	2GB RAM, 2GHz processor	27	29	31
Dell Inspiron XPS M1310	2GB RAM, 1.6GHz processor	36	39	48
Hp pavilion dv 200	2GB RAM, 2GHz processor	34	41	42
Fujitsu Siemens AMILO M7440	512 MB RAM, 1.73GHz processor	29	31	35
Lenovo ThinkPad X60	512 MB RAM, 1.6 GHz processor	21	25	28

3.1 Laptops

We looked at nine different laptop models belonging to various manufacturers and measured their power consumption. Since communication is an integral part of portable computing devices, we paid special attention to the state of the wireless network interface card (WNIC). We kept the laptops in three different states: Idle with WNIC off, Idle with WNIC on (but no traffic sent or received), and receiving streaming video through WNIC. All laptops were running Windows XP or Vista, and were measured when idling with no applications running. By averaging the "Idle with WNIC on" column in Table 1, factoring in some additional power for traffic, we arrive at an average consumption of a laptop around 35 W, with some approximation.

Similar numbers have been reported by prior studies with laptops [22, 23]. These studies also provided the power breakdown across different components of a laptop. We show this breakdown in Figure 2 for the sake of completeness of this paper. It can be seen that, for an active laptop, about

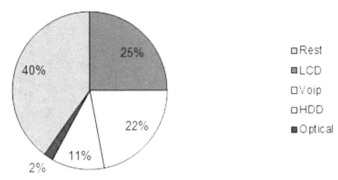

Figure 2 Power consumption breakdown of a laptop making VoIP calls.

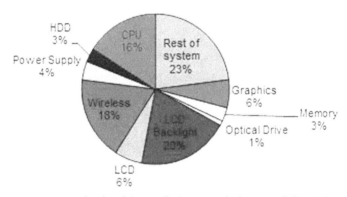

Figure 3 Power consumption breakdown of a laptop actively transmitting FTP traffic [22].

20% of the power consumption is due to the WNIC and rivals power consumption due to the display and CPU. As the work and results by Mahesri and Vardhan [22] (shown in Figure 3) is based on currently outdated hardware, we did our own study of the energy consumed by different components of a Lenovo SL400 laptop during a Voice over IP (VoIP) call which is a popular application. Our results (Figure 2) show that the network interface is still a significant consumer of energy compared to the LCD, CPU, memory, and other components.

3.2 Mobile Phones

Our study of mobile phone power consumption was based on only one smartphone, the Samsung BlackJack, which does not have a Wi-Fi WNIC. The Bluetooth interface was kept off. The idle phone consumed about 1 W while during a call it consumed 3 W. Thus, during active communication, the communication interface consumes about two-thirds the power of the device. This is confirmed by other studies done on devices with Wi-Fi interfaces like PDA's [24]. Studies by Nokia also confirm that mobile phones typically take little more than 1 W of power on average (1.2 W to be precise).

Since all emerging smartphones like the Apple iPhone and RIM Black-berry have a Wi-Fi interface in addition to the cellular interface, we believe our estimate of power consumption of mobile phones is a conservative one.

4 Accounting for Number of Portable Devices

In this section we account for the number of portable computing devices used in the world. As before, we focus on only two classes: laptops and mobile phones. Based on the cumulative numbers determined in this section, coupled with the power consumed for each of these devices as presented in the previous section, we will account for global energy consumed due to portable devices annually in the following section.

4.1 Laptops

Based on the total computing numbers reported in Section 2, our challenge here is to identify the number of laptops from this overall projected number of computers in the world. Recent trends have shown that mobile computing is the most rapidly expanding segment in the computer industry. Historically laptops always have cost more than their desk counterparts. With advancements in microelectronics and continuing validity of Moore's Law, laptops are becoming cheap and affordable. Advancements in Wi-Fi technology are making mobile connectivity more and more ubiquitous, and one of the biggest factors driving the popularity of laptop computers. With ever increasing processing speed and lower costs, more and more people prefer laptops. One of the watershed events in the history of computers was achieved in 2008 when the number of laptops sold exceeded those of desktops for the first time [25]. According to an International Data Corporation (IDC) survey, the third quarter of 2008 saw notebook shipments into the US market surpass 50% of the share of the computer market. The figure for laptops stood at 55.2% as per IDC's US Quarterly PC Tracker [26]. It becomes abundantly clear from the above studies that laptops (and devices like tablets of similar form factor) are increasingly preferred and their ratio is set to increase in the future as people becomes more mobile. For our study we can estimate the number of laptops currently in use to be around 460 million based on numbers presented in Section 2 and current market share and projected trends.

4.2 Mobile Phones

Mobile communication is one of the most rapidly expanding technologies has influenced every facet of human life since its inception. Thanks to the economic viability and decreasing prices of micro-electronic components, more people are able to own a mobile phone than ever before. When it comes to electricity consumption, we have reached a stage where mobile phones and related telecommunication infrastructure can no longer be ignored anymore because of their sheer volume. At the end of 2008, an important milestone in the ICT development race was achieved with over 4 billion mobile cellular subscriptions worldwide [27, 28].

Similarly the number of more sophisticated and processing oriented mobile phones is on rise. It is estimated that the number of smart-phones sold in five years will triple reaching 60 million [29]. Among the top 25 growth markets ranking list (2006–2011) there are a few surprises. India wins the top spot, just ahead of China, and almost equally in third place are Brazil, Indonesia, and Nigeria, but the real surprises start in the sixth place with the US mobile market tipped to grow by almost 66 million net additions from the start of 2006 to the end of 2011 [30]. The latest figures suggest that 5 billion mobile phones are in circulation [31] so we can estimate the total number of mobile phones globally to be 5 billion.

5 Energy Consumed by Personal Computing in Global Perspective

In this section we account for global energy consumption and focus specifically on the overall electricity consumed. By calculating the energy used for various segments of computing devices, we subsequently show the energy consumed by computing devices as a percentage of global electricity consumption. Furthermore, we specifically characterize what percentage of the computing segment is consumed by portable devices alone.

5.1 Global Figures

According to the World Energy Outlook-2008 Executive Summary published by International Energy Agency, global primary energy demand will increase

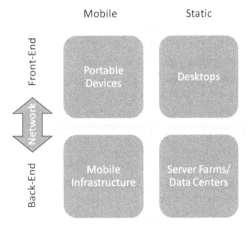

Figure 4 Elements considered in our definition of personal computing.

at an average of 1.6% per annum from 2006 to 2030. In 2006 the total energy consumption was estimated to be 11,730 million tones of oil equivalent (Mtoe) which is projected to increase to 17,010 Mtoe by 2030 [32]. Using above estimates, the approximate energy consumption in 2010 translates to 145 trillion KWh. Now the next step will be to approximate the total amount of electricity consumed globally. According to Central Intelligence Agency (CIA) World Factbook estimates, the amount of electricity consumed worldwide in 2008 was around 16.88 trillion KWh [33]. Using this amount, and assuming a modest 3% increase in global electricity consumption, the overall number for 2010 can be estimated as 17.8 trillion KWh indicating that electricity is about 12% of global energy consumption.

5.2 Computing Figures Including Portable Devices

Next, we will try to account for the approximate energy consumption by various front-end and back-end elements of the personal computing segment as defined in Figure 4, including those of the network infrastructure that connects them.

5.2.1 Energy Consumption by Portable Devices

According to our earlier estimates 5 billion mobile phones are currently used world-wide. Annual electricity consumption for a mobile phone as cited by the Nokia study is around 11 KWh per year [34], or around 1.2 W per unit at a given time. This figure is confirmed by our calculations with smart-phones in Section 3. The annual energy consumption of all mobile devices in the world can thus be estimated at 55 million MWh.

Based on our earlier discussion, we estimate the number of laptops in the world to be approximately around 460 million. Average power consumed by a single laptop is about 35 W [23]. We assume that a laptop is used about ten hours a day, therefore the energy consumption of a single laptop for a year is around 127.7 KWh. Hence overall energy consumption in the world due to usage of all the laptops would be around 58 Million MWh.

5.2.2 Energy Consumption by Desktop Computers

From our assumptions in Section 2.3, there are about 1000 million desktop computers. The average power consumption of a 'typical' desktop is about 150 W based on a study by Intel [23], which includes the power consumed by a 17-inch LCD monitor. That study notes that without the LCD monitor, the system power consumption would be about 65 W.

We assume that an average desktop PC is used for about eight hours a day so that the energy consumption of one desktop computer with LCD display used for a year with an average power 150 W is about 438 KWh. Hence, 1000 million desktop computers consume about 438 million MWh annually. This is a conservative estimate, which does not take into account those desktops that are active or left idle for 24 hours a day.

5.2.3 Energy Consumption by Data Centers

From our earlier discussion in Section 2, electricity consumed globally by data centers during operation is 175 million MWh. This figure is the energy consumed during the operation of the computing equipment in datacenters. This does not include the energy needed for cooling and power distribution which was estimated to be roughly equivalent to the energy cost of computation in [9]. Since this article's focus is on the computation aspects and how more efficient computing techniques can reduce energy consumption, we do not show the cooling and power distribution energy consumption except in Section 7 where we compare energy consumed for the personal computing segment from a lifecycle perspective, including all energy costs during the period of usage. A discussion on achieving efficiency in cooling and power distribution is out of scope of this article.

5.2.4 Energy Consumption for Mobile Infrastructure

According to the Ericsson study [19], mobile communications infrastructure (including lifecycle costs and mobile handsets) consumed about 0.12% of energy globally in 2007. We can budgeting for a 15–20% increase over this share for the year 2010 to avoid an underestimate resulting in a share of 0.14%.[2]

Taking into account that only 53% of the above figure is consumed as electricity during actual operation [19] and global energy consumption is 145 trillion KWh, the electricity consumed for mobile communications infrastructure (including mobile handset operation) can be estimated as 107 million MWh. Subtracting the electricity consumed by mobile handsets as found above of 55 million MWh, we can estimate the mobile infrastructure consumes 52 million MWh. The study in [19] was mainly for GSM base stations and not 3G and 4G base-stations that are being rolled out. However, the presentation in [57] points out that these new base stations consume comparable power, allowing us to use the above estimate.

5.2.5 Internet/Computer Networks

With a large number of people in developing countries joining the IT revolution, the energy required keep networks, including routers, switches, and firewalls running is becoming quite considerable. The above mentioned study [10] estimated this amount to be 219 million MWh in 2008. Since the Internet is greatly expanding fueled by the ever increasing demand of more and more data, multimedia, online gaming and new applications, and extrapolating the growth patterns from [10] we can estimate the overall energy consumption in 2010 to be around 300 million MWh. We introduce this number along with other elements of personal computing to provide a complete perspective.

Figure 5 shows how the energy consumed by portable devices compares with that of other elements of personal computing. Traditionally, data centers and mobile infrastructures have been considered as the power hogs within the ICT area, and most prior work in energy efficiency has specifically targeted only these two areas [35–41]. However, the results above show that personal computing devices consume comparable if not more energy and it is worthwhile to research ways to achieve energy-efficient operation for these as well.

---

[2] We prefer to overestimate energy consumption for the mobile infrastructure when there is some uncertainty as this prevents the overall share due to personal computing from being an overestimate as well.

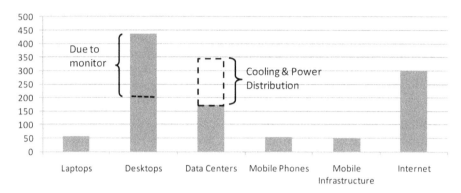

Figure 5 Comparison of energy consumed by portable devices with other elements of personal computing.

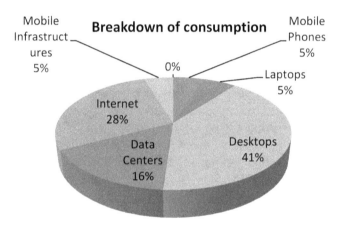

Figure 6 Personal computing related electricity vs. global electricity use.

5.3 Personal Computing in Global Perspective

From the above calculations, we can obtain an estimate for total electricity consumed by personal computing devices. The combined electricity consumed by the entire computation sector for 2010 was 1078 million MWh. Hence, electricity consumed by computational devices is 6% of the global electricity consumption. Figure 6 shows the segment-wise percentage contribution while Figure 7 illustrates the ICT electricity consumption vs. global electricity consumption.

ICT electricity vs total electricity

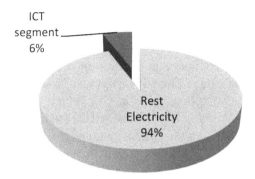

Figure 7 Global electricity consumption vs. total ICT sector electricity consumption.

Portable sector vs overall ICT

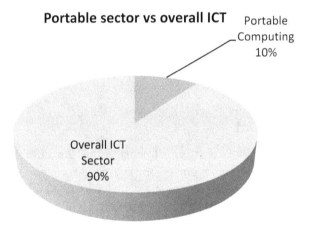

Figure 8 Total personal computing sector electricity use vs. portable sector.

From the above-mentioned numbers, we can also calculate the individual contribution of portable devices versus the whole computation segment. Overall consumption is 1078 million MWh whereas the contribution of the portable segment (including only laptops and mobile phones) is 107 million MWh. Hence, portable devices contribute close to 10% of the energy consumed by computational devices. This contribution is further elaborated in Figure 8. As we deduced, the contribution of electricity to the overall global energy sector is about 12%. From our numbers, we can also ascertain the contribution of the computation sector to the overall global energy consumption as a modest 0.71%.

5.4 Limitations

The readers should make note that some of the numbers presented are estimates based on available data. There is expected to be some variability based on source of data and assumptions made by that source. For example, we used a value of 2 for Power Usage Effectiveness (PUE) from [9] for data centers that represents the ratio of energy costs for running the data center to the energy cost for just computing operations. It could be the case that some data centers operate with a lower PUE than this. Other examples include assumptions on average usage durations for various computing devices. As all our accounting numbers and methodology is described fully in this article, we expect the readers to be able to modify our calculations as needed when more accurate data is available for an particular segment. It should also be easy to extend our results for additional years as new data becomes available. We expect that in future tablet computers and smart phones and their impact would need to be incorporated.

6 Broader Impact

In this section we look at other dimensions of the numbers obtained in Section 5 and earlier. We begin by presenting the energy consumption by computing devices in terms of carbon di-oxide (CO_2) emissions to demonstrate environmental impact. Subsequently, we will look at the amount of residential electricity consumption by computing devices to get a consumer perspective as well.

6.1 Environmental Impact

One of the major points that often remain unnoticed is that, although electrical energy consumption represents only 12% of the global energy requirements, its contribution to the global CO_2 emissions is a whopping 40%. A study by International Energy Agency entitled CO_2 emissions by sectors released in 2005 puts the CO_2 emissions worldwide due to public electricity and heating to 37.2% [42]. Similar studies by European Commission's Directorate-General for Energy and Transport released in 2009 for the year 2006 puts the CO_2 emissions in the European Union (EU) zone because of energy industries and household to be around 48% [43]. Surprisingly, coal is still one of the major fuels employed to generate electricity worldwide. For example according to American Coal Foundation about 56% of electricity generated in the US is done through coal [44]. Based on report on CO_2 emissions by different power plants in the US by Energy Information Administration, for every kWh of electricity generation, 2.117 pounds of CO_2 is produced by burning coal, 1.915 pounds from petroleum and 1.314 pounds from gas [45, 46]. Hence on average electricity sources emit 1.297 lbs CO_2 per kWh (0.0005883 metric tons CO_2 per kWh). Thus, given that 1078 million MWh is contributed by the personal computing segment, it responsible for about 0.63 billion tons of CO_2 annually. One way to interpret this is that it is equivalent to the emissions of 10.35 million vehicles on the road when driving 10,000 miles per year considering an average car giving 21 miles per gallon (mpg). Another way to interpret this is that these emissions are equivalent to 0.5 KWh per day per capita, or every person on the planet running a 1 KW electric heater, 30 minutes a day throughout the year. The consideration of source of energy is interesting as well. 73% of emissions in the electricity generation sector come solely from coal which explains why this sector has disproportionately high level of CO_2 emissions as compared to other segments; even though the computing sector electricity consumption is only 0.71% of the global energy consumption, this fragment contributes to 2% of global CO_2 emissions as illustrated in Figure 9 [7, 48]. *Therefore the computing sector presents a very attractive opportunity in the global race to control greenhouse emissions.*[3]

6.2 Individual Consumer Perspective

As per the US Department of Energy [49], energy consumption per household in the US for a year is about 11000 KWh. The average number of people per household is about 2.59 as per the US Census Bureau [50]. Assuming that there will soon be (if not already) two mobile phones, one desktop and one laptop in a typical home, the total energy cost due to computing would be around 580 KWh using our calculations in Section 5. The corresponding energy consumption due to only portable devices (one laptop and two mobile phones) would be around 150 KWh. Hence, energy consumption due to computing in an average residential home in the US would be around 5.25% while energy consumption due to portable devices would be about 1.36%.

---

[3] Of course, cleaning up electricity generation itself is an useful goal that has broad consensus among the research community with various efforts underway, but is outside the scope of this paper.

Contribution of ICT CO2 emissions

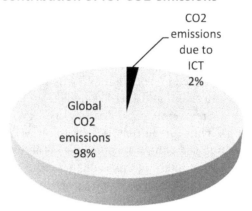

Figure 9 Global CO_2 emissions due to ICT sector vs. global CO_2 emissions.

To get another viewpoint we also consider the statistics of one of the rapidly growing economies in the world: India. The domestic energy consumption in India was 20.8 Mtoe in 1990 and about 56.5 Mtoe in 2001. Based on projected rate of growth, we estimate that the domestic energy consumption in 2009 would be around 82.46 Mtoe that is roughly equivalent to 0.959 trillion KWh. The population of India as per World Statesmen [51] is about 1.14 billion. Considering there are 4.8 people per household [51], the average household energy consumption would be 4038 KWh. With 2 mobile phones, 1 laptop, and 1 desktop per household as above,[4] the share of energy consumption due to computing would be 14.36%, while that of portable devices would be 3.71%. These numbers are presented in Figure 10.

Hence it can be observed that in developing economies like India, the computing device energy consumption share is much higher due to general household energy consumption being lower compared to the US.

---

[4] This assumption holds typically in urban areas in India, but in rural areas only the assumption of 2 mobile phones is justified with far fewer laptops and desktops [52, 53]. Nevertheless, these numbers are projected to be true in the very near future as most of India's middle-class already had at least one desktop or laptop by 2006 [17, 54]. Thus, for ease of comparison, we keep the number of household computing devices to be the same both in India and the US. Note that there are more people per household on average in India than the US, and thus, the former could be considered to have a greater potential to utilize more computing devices per household in the future.

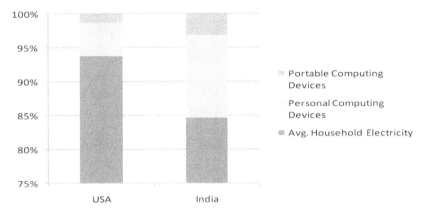

Figure 10 Comparison of household electricity consumption due to personal computing devices in the US and India. Note that the Y-axis starts at 75% to clearly show relative percentage differences.

7 Recommendations for Energy-Efficient, Sustainable Portable Computing

The issue of energy consumption of computing devices can best be alleviated by all members of the computing community that include researchers working on different aspects like displays, CPUs, network interfaces, memory, to talk of a few. Individual optimizations to each hardware component would help, and could be improved by joint hardware optimizations. Similarly, software optimizations focusing on operating systems, data caching, data compression, to name a few, would be helpful as studied, and even put into practice over the last decade or so. In this section, we pay particular attention on how to reduce energy consumed by portable devices.

We believe that computer networking researchers can contribute the most in reducing portable device energy consumption due to the fact that an active network interface is likely to be the task that consumes the most power among all components, as seen in Section 3. Our following recommendations are thus aimed directly at the networking community, including possible cross-component approaches.

We classify our recommendations into two categories: energy-efficient operation, and increasing lifespan. The first category deals with how to design and/or operate a device more efficiently. The second category deals with how to decrease the energy costs based on a lifecycle approach, primarily focusing on reducing the impact of manufacturing by increasing lifespan.

7.1 Energy-Efficient Operation

7.1.1 Power Management

Power management has been an active area of research over the years for computing devices as well as appliances [13]. Device components have been optimized to lower power consumption. There are at least two areas where further work can be done apart from continued optimizations of components individually.

The *first area* is to make users utilize power management more often. An informal survey of 50 students at our university showed that most were unaware of power management modes of the network card, and used the default settings. A simple check of the default settings of laptops studied in Section 3 earlier showed that power management was disabled by default.

The *second area*, once users are aware of power management options, is to enable tunable software based trade-offs between energy and performance. For example, wireless cards can be kept in sleep mode longer at the expense of higher delay of received packets, for, say, a VoIP application [58]. Or, the resolution of a video being streamed could be reduced for reduced energy consumption [59]. The creation of a general framework across different computing platforms to allow such tunable tradeoffs is sorely required. If the hardware equivalent of a 'knob' could be developed that allows each users to tune it to their own tolerable performance levels, it would make power management more acceptable.

7.1.2 Battery Management

When batteries are necessary, as is the case when a user is mobile, better usage of batteries can get better efficiencies. Protocols and algorithms should be designed to provide time for battery charge recovery, and use less current draw when possible. For example, medium access control (or even upper layer) protocols could be designed that send and receive packets in short bursts, that allows nodes enough time in sleep mode in between bursts [55]. Greater utilization of battery capacity can reduce power consumed of the electricity grid.

7.1.3 Adjust Optimization Metrics

Protocols and algorithms should be designed keeping total energy consumption as a metric, as opposed to individual node lifetimes when considering a collaborative network in specific scenarios. For example, consider the case of a static wireless mesh network. It may be possible to replace the batteries in such nodes periodically. In such an instance, protocols must be designed to minimize total energy consumption of the network as opposed to each node trying to minimize its energy consumption [56]. Another example is that of an ad hoc network in a conference room where a power outlet for each node is easily available and all nodes are plugged in. Again, in this scenario, the total power consumption by all nodes should be minimized as opposed to the common metric of individual node consumption.

7.1.4 Utilize Energy Harvesting

Recently, there are many products on the market which allow the use of energy harvesting techniques to power portable devices. For example, the Solaris product (cost about $360) from Brunton can charge laptops, while the SolarPort product (cost $120) from the same manufacturer can charge smaller devices like phones. These devices can become more main-stream with time as prices drop due to scale, or through government subsidies to encourage more renewable energy use. Of course, one must also weigh the energy benefits of solar panels against the actual energy needed to manufacture them.

From a networking researcher's perspective, there is a need to understand how to design protocols to utilize such sources of energy effectively. For example, during periods when plenty of energy is available, portable devices could do more of delay-tolerant tasks. Once the energy harvest is unavailable, the device can ramp down to minimal operating modes similar to the power management paradigm.

7.2 Increasing Lifespan

There are two approaches which could result in consumers using their devices longer: economic incentives, and reliance on thin-client paradigms.

The first approach could be to provide economic incentives for consumers, or at least remove the current incentives to stop using phones after a period of time. For example, typical cellular phone carrier contracts in the US last for two years after which customers typically upgrade to newer devices that are heavily subsidized conditional on the signing of a two-year contract. If consumers would instead buy hardware without contracts and subsidies, they might be inclined to keep their devices longer. As reducing energy consumed for manufacturing devices and decreasing environmental waste provides environmental benefits, governments could provide incentives for consumers to keep their devices. For example, the government could pay a part of carrier costs after a device has been used over a period of time. Note that, typically governments and manufacturers would prefer consumers to keep buying and replacing their phones. Thus, in this case the services and software aspect of maintaining or improving user satisfaction would need to be encouraged more than replacing hardware, apart from the incentives mentioned above.

The second approach could be to rely more on a thin-client paradigm where individual consumer devices would have reduced capabilities acting as 'dumb' terminals with most of the processing done at remote servers. This would allow most upgrades to be done at the servers, with little incentive for consumers to upgrade their devices. This approach would require greater reliance on software upgrades than hardware upgrades. There is likely to be an increased burden on communication within the thin-client paradigm which would then need the design of energy-efficient communication techniques.

Additional approaches could include greater modularity in the way portable communication devices are manufactured so that, with the replacement of only a few parts, desired functionality can be maintained. Currently available devices, especially mobile phones, are rarely modular with the whole device needing replacement with the malfunction of one of the major components. This should be an additional area of research towards the quest for sustainability in portable computing and communication devices.

8 Conclusions

We presented a revised and updated study over [60] that accounted for energy consumed by various computing devices, including the growing portable device segment. In [60] our key results were that ICT accounted for only 3% of global electricity consumption with portable devices responsible for 17% of this share. In this updated study including electricity consumption due to the Internet infrastructure, our accounting shows that computing consumes about 6% of the global electricity consumption. Of this, about 10% is contributed by portable devices, still a significantly high share. This statistic should serve as a reminder to researchers that energy should also be treated as a resource consumption issue in portable computing devices, as opposed to the traditional operating lifetime metric. Our study also shows that the CO_2 emissions due to the computing sector are much higher due to the fuel source used for power, and efficiencies in the computing sector can make a bigger impact on global CO_2 emissions than efficient practices in other sectors. From an individual consumer perspective, we also demonstrate that the cost of electricity for computing rivals that of many other common household appliances, and requires careful thought on usage behavior. This is especially true in developing countries like India where average household energy consumption is lower than the US, and results in the share of computing devices being higher. We made specific recommendations for greater energy-efficiency and sustainability in the portable computing area through a combination of reduction of energy consumption during the use phase, and increase in lifespan through economic incentives and reliance on thin-client paradigms.

References

[1] G. Fettweis and E. Zimmermann. ICT Energy Consumption – Trends and Challenges in Proceedings of the 11th International Symposium on Wireless Personal Multimedia Communications (WPMC'08), Lapland, Finland, 08–11 September 2008.
[2] Carrie A. Webber, Judy A. Roberson, Marla C. McWhinney, Richard E. Brown, Margaret J. Pinckard, and John F. Busch. After-hours power status of office equipment in the USA. *Energy*, 31:2487–2502, 2006.
[3] Kaoru Kawamoto, Yoshiyuki Shimoda, and Minoru Mizuno. Energy saving potential of office equipment power management. *Energy and Buildings*, 36:915–923, 2004.
[4] U. Hölzle. Powering a Google Search. Official Google Blog, January 2009.
[5] A. Qureshi, R. Weber et al. Cutting the electric bill for internet-scale systems. In *Proceedings SIGCOMM'09*, Barcelona, Spain, August 17–21, 2009.
[6] Report to Congress on Server and Data Center Energy Efficiency Public Law 109-431, EPA ENERGY STAR Program, 2 August 2007.
[7] Data Center Energy Savings, available at http://perfectsearchcorp.com/data-center-energy-savings.
[8] Gartner: Data Centres Account for 23% of Global ICT CO2 Emissions, 5 November 2007, available online at http://engineers.ihs.com/news/gartner-datacentre-co2.htm.
[9] J.G. Koomey. Worldwide electricity used in data centers. *Environmental Research Letters*, 3, 2008.
[10] M. Pickavet, W. Vereecken, S. Demeyer, P. Audenaert, B. Vermeulen, C. Develder, D. Colle, B. Dhoedt, and P. Demeester. Worldwide energy needs for ICT: The rise of power-aware networking. In *Proceedings IEEE ANTS 2008 Conference*, Bombay (India), 15–17 December 2008.
[11] US Department of Energy. Annual energy outlook 2005 with projections to 2025. Energy Information Administration, Washington, DC, DOE/EIA-0383 (2005), 2005.
[12] C.A. Webber, R.E. Brown, and J.G. Koomey. Savings estimates for the Energy Star voluntary labeling program. *Energy Policy*, 28:1137–1149, 2000.
[13] R. Brown, C. Webber, and J.G. Koomey. Status and future directions of the Energy Star program. *Energy*, 27:505–520, 2002.

[14] Energy Star® Overview of 2008 achievements, http://www.energystar.gov/ia/partners/publications/pubdocs/2008%204%20pager%203-12-09.pdf.

[15] The green shoots of hi-tech success, report available at http://news.bbc.co.uk/2/hi/technology/6983117.stm.

[16] Annual Forecast Statements 1993–2009, Computer Industry Almanac Inc., available at http://www.c-i-a.com/.

[17] Press Release, Forrester Research Inc., available at http://www.forrester.com/ER/Press/Release/0,1769,1151,00.html.

[18] Gartner says more than 1 billion PCs in use worldwide and headed to 2 billion units by 2014, Press Release, available at http://www.gartner.com/it/page.jsp?id=703807.

[19] Sustainable energy use in mobile communications. White Paper by Ericsson, August 2007.

[20] Iceland looks to serve the world, report available at http://news.bbc.co.uk/2/hi/programmes/click_online/8297237.stm.

[21] Kill-A-Watt Meter, online available at http://www.p3international.com/products/special/P4400/P4400-CE.html.

[22] Aqeel Mahesri and Vibhore Vardhan. Power consumption breakdown on a modern laptop. In *Proceedings of Workshop on Power Aware Computing Systems, 37th International Symposium on Microarchitecture (PACS)*, December 2004.

[23] Intel Corporation, PC Energy-Efficiency Trends and Technologies, online available at cache-www.intel.com/cd/00/00/10/27/102727_ar024103.pdf.

[24] Vijay Raghunathan, Trevor Pering, Roy Want, Alex Nguyen, and Peter Jensen. Experience with a low power wireless mobile computing platform. In *Proceedings of the 2004 International Symposium on Low Power Electronics and Design (ISLPED'04)*, pp. 363–368, 2004.

[25] Notebook PC shipments exceed desktops for first time in Q3, iSuppli applied market intelligence, Press Report, available at http://www.isuppli.com/News/Pages/Notebook-PC-Shipments-Exceed-Desktops-for-First-Time-in-Q3.aspx?.

[26] Notebook shipments surpass desktops in the US market for the first time, IDC Press Release, available at http://www.idc.com/getdoc.jsp?containerId=prUS22383910 (accessed January 18, 2011).

[27] Measuring the Information Society, The ICT Development Index, International Telecommunications Union Society, 2009.

[28] Mark Walsh. US mobile broadband users to surpass 140 million by 2013. January 6, 2009, available at http://www.mediapost.com/publications/.

[29] Half the world will use a mobile phone by 2009, available at http://www.cellular-news.com/story/15674.php.

[30] Half world's population 'will have mobile phone by end of year' online news article available at http://www.guardian.co.uk/technology/2008/sep/26/mobilephones.unitednations.

[31] CNET Reviews, Cell phone subscriptions to hit 5 billion globally, available at http://reviews.cnet.com/8301-13970_7-10454065-78.html, accessed July 2010.

[32] World Energy Outlook 2008, Executive Summary, International Energy Agency, available online at http://www.iea.org/weo/docs/weo2008/WEO2008_es_English.pdf.

[33] CIA World Factbook, Annual Report, available at http://www.indexmundi.com/world/electricity_consumption.html.

[34] Report by Nokia. Online available at http://ec.europa.eu/environment/ipp/pdf/nokia_mobile_05_04.pdf.

[35] P. Ranganathan. Recipe for efficiency: principles of power-aware computing. *Commun. ACM*, 53(4):60–67, 2010.

[36] J. Loper and S. Parr. Energy efficiency in data centers: A new policy frontier. *Environmental Quality Management*, 16(4):83–97, June 2007.

[37] N. Laoutaris, P. Rodriguez, and L. Massoulie. Echos: edge capacity hosting overlays of nano data centers. *SIGCOMM Comput. Commun. Rev.*, 38(1):51–54, 2008.

[38] C. Lefurgy, K. Rajamani, F. Rawson, W. Felter, M. Kistler, and T. W. Keller. Energy management for commercial servers. *Computer*, 36(12):39–48, 2003.

[39] Y. Chen, A. Das, W. Qin, A. Sivasubramaniam, Q. Wang, and N. Gautam, Managing server energy and operational costs in hosting centers. *SIGMETRICS Perform. Eval. Rev.*, 33(1):303–314, 2005.

[40] V. Bassoo, K. Tom, A. K. Mustafa, E. Cijvat, H. Sjoland, and M. Faulkner. A potential transmitter architecture for future generation green wireless base station. *EURASIP J. Wirel. Commun. Netw.*, 2009:2–10, 2009.

[41] Ericsson. Sustainable energy use in mobile communications, August 2007, http://www.ericsson.com/campaign/.

[42] Carbon Dioxide Emissions by Economic Sector 2005, Report by International Energy Agency.

[43] CO_2 Emissions by Sector, EU ENERGY IN FIGURES 2009, Report by Directorate-General for Energy and Transport, European Commission.

[44] FAQs about coal, American Coal Foundation available at http://www.teachcoal.org/aboutcoal/articles/faqs.html.

[45] Carbon Dioxide Emissions from the Generation of Electric Power in the United States, report available at http://www.eia.doe.gov/cneaf/electricity/page/co2_report/co2emiss.pdf.

[46] Report from Carbonfund. Available online at http://www.carbonfund.org/site/pages/carbon_calculators/category/Assumptions.

[47] Power Scorecard, Electricity from coal available online at
http://www.powerscorecard.org/tech_detail.cfm?resource_id=2.

[48] World CO_2 Emissions to Rise 75 Pct by 2030 – EIA, at http://www.planetark.com/dailynewsstory.cfm/newsid/36924/story.htm.

[49] Energy savers, US Department of Energy. Retrieved from http://www1.eere.energy.gov/consumer/tips/appliances.html.

[50] Quick facts, US Census Bureau, retrieved from http://quickfacts.census.gov/qfd/states/00000.html.

[51] World Population Trends, World Statesmen Forum, retrieved from, http://www.worldstatesmen.org/India.htm.

[52] Average Residential Energy Consumption per Household, retrieved from http://www.nfhsindia.org/ on October 23, 2009.

[53] Telecom Regulatory Authority of India (TRAI) Annual Report available online at http://www.trai.gov.in/annualreport/TRAIAR2008-09E.pdf.

[54] Wired Generation, India Today, available online at http://www.india-today.com/itoday/20061120/cover.html.

[55] C.F. Chiasserini and R.R. Rao, Pulsed battery discharge in communication devices. In *Proceedings of the 5th Annual ACM/IEEE International Conference on Mobile Computing and Networking*, Seattle, Washington, August 15–19, pp. 88–95, 1999.

[56] Vinod Namboodiri, Lixin Gao, and Ramakrishna Janaswamy. Power efficient topology control for wireless networks with switched beam directional antennas. *Elsevier Ad Hoc Networks*, 6(2), April 2008.

[57] P. Grant, Green Radio C. The case for more efficient cellular base stations, University of Edinburgh, 2009. Online available at http://www.see.ed.ac.uk/∼ pmg/green_radio.ppt, accessed January 18, 2011.

[58] Y. Agarwal, R. Chandra, A. Wolman, P. Bahl, K. Chin, and R. Gupta. Wireless wakeups revisited: Energy management for VoIP over Wi-Fi smartphones. In *Proceedings ACM/USENIX MobiSys*, 2007.

[59] P. Shenoy and P. Radkov. Proxy-assisted power-friendly streaming to mobile devices. In *Proceedings of MMCN*, 2003.

[60] P. Somavat, S. Jadhav, and V. Namboodiri. Accounting for the energy consumption of personal computing including portable devices. In *Proceedings of the 1st International Conference on Energy-Efficient Computing and Networking (e-Energy)*, Passau, Germany, pp. 141–149, April 2010.

Biographies

Pavel Somavat is currently working as Assistant Professor in Electrical Engineering at CCS Haryana Agricultural University, India. He obtained his M.S. in Information & Communications Engineering from University of Applied Sciences Giessen Friedberg, Friedberg, Germany. He has worked as a researcher in fiber optics industry working in the field of dynamic attenuation testing on fibers. His research interests are diverse ranging from energy efficiency issues in ICT sector to optical fiber based sensors. He has published work in estimating the environmental effects of rapid proliferation of ICT technologies and the probable directions for ensuring sustainable development.

Vinod Namboodiri is currently Assistant Professor at the Department of Electrical Engineering and Computer Science at Wichita State University, USA. He graduated with a Ph.D. in Electrical and Computer engineering from the University of Massachusetts Amherst in 2008. He has served or is currently serving on the technical program committees of IEEE GLOBE-COM, IEEE ICC, IEEE IPCCC, and IEEE GREENCOM, and is an active reviewer for numerous journals and conferences in the wireless networking and mobile computing areas. His research interests include designing algorithms and protocols for energy-intelligent and sustainable computing, and designing an effective communication architecture for smart electric grids. In the past he has worked on designed MAC and routing protocols, and developing energy-efficient protocols and algorithms for different wireless technologies like Wireless LANs, RFID Systems, Wireless Sensor Networks, and Wireless Mesh Networks.

Analysis of Power Consumption in OFDM Systems

Irena Orović, Nikola Žarić, Srdjan Stanković, Igor Radusinović and
Zoran Veljović

*Faculty of Electrical Engineering, University of Montenegro, 20000 Podgorica,
Montenegro; e-mail: zaric@ac.me*

Received: 8 July 2011; Accepted: 21 July 2011

Abstract

The energy efficiency of various OFDM systems, such as optical, mobile,
Wireless and WiMaX systems, has been analyzed in this paper. High peak to
average power ratio that may appear in modulation process is one of the main
problems in OFDM systems. The influence of subcarriers number and modulation techniques to the peak-to-average power ratio in different OFDM based
systems has been studied. The results of analysis are presented in numerous
figures and tables. The main goal is to provide a comparative study that can
be used for an optimal system selection with predefined power consumption
requirements.

Keywords: OFDM, peak-to-average power ratio, transmission systems.

1 Introduction

Orthogonal frequency division multiplexing (OFDM) provides transmission
of multiple signals simultaneously over a single transmission path. Each
signal is transmitted within its own frequency range (carrier), which is modulated by the data symbols. This technique provides high data rate even if
relatively small frequency bandwidth is available. Also, OFDM based system
has other favorable properties such as high spectral efficiency, robustness to

Journal of Green Engineering, 477–489.

channel fading and impulse interference [1, 2]. Therefore, OFDM has been used in numerous modern transmission systems, as for example, in Wireless IEEE 802.11a/g/n/e, digital audio broadcasting, digital video broadcasting (satellite, terrestrial, cable), fixed and mobile WiMaX, etc.

On the other hand, the OFDM systems are characterized by high peak-to-average power ratio (PAPR) [3–11]. A large PAPR appears as a consequence of the multicarrier OFDM signal nature. Namely, adding all carriers together can result in high maximum peak power, which can further increase with the number of carriers. For signals having large PAPR, the problem may appear during amplification at the transmitter. High signal values can be non-linearly amplified due to the small dynamic range of the amplifier, which will cause signal distortions. In order to avoid distortions, the mean signal power should be decreased, which then leads to a high power consumption and a low amplifier efficiency. Having in mind that the low power consumption is an important requirement in modern communication systems (e.g. in mobile systems), significant efforts have been made to develop techniques that are able to reduce PAPR [4–11].

In this paper we have analyzed the influence of subcarriers number to the PAPR for various OFDM based systems. Also, the influence of modulation techniques to the PAPR has been discussed. Further, we have considered different PAPR reduction techniques, as well as, their performances in different OFDM systems. A comparative analysis of these techniques is provided, which can be useful for optimal system selection.

2 OFDM Systems – Theoretical Background

OFDM based systems have been introduced to improve performances of previously used conventional transmission systems such as time division multiplex and frequency division multiplex based systems. High data transmission rates, high spectral efficiency, robustness, simple implementation are some of the characteristics that recommend OFDM as a standard for almost all modern communication systems

The block scheme of an OFDM system is shown in Figure 1. The input data sequence is usually processed with some digital modulator, such as BPSK, QPSK, 4QAM, 16QAM, 64QAM, etc. The choice of modulation technique significantly influences the data transmission rate. For example, if 16QAM is used, the transmission rate will be 8 times higher than if BPSK is used. However, the PAPR will be also significantly higher in the case of 16QAM, which will be discussed in the next section.

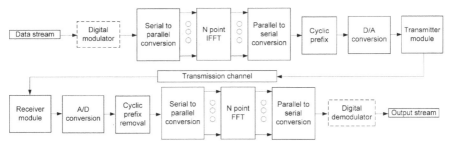

Figure 1   General block scheme of OFDM system.

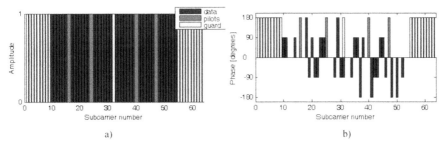

a)   b)

Figure 2   Frequency domain representation of one OFDM symbol: (a) amplitude of subcarriers, (b) phase of subcarriers.

The modulated sequence is converted into K parallel low bit rate data streams, where K represents the number of subcarriers used for data transmission. Each data stream is assigned to the appropriate subcarrier as follows:

$$s_k(t) = A_k e^{(2j\pi f_k t + \phi_k)}, \tag{1}$$

where A_k and φ_k are parameters of modulated symbol, while f_k represents the subcarrier frequency. The amplitude and phase representation of modulated subcarriers (in the case of QPSK modulation) for one OFDM symbol are shown in Figure 2. Note that, in this example, only $K = 40$ subcarriers are used to transmit data, while the remaining subcarriers are reserved for pilot symbols (4 subcarriers) and guard intervals (19 subcarriers). Also, having in mind properties of Fourier transform, the DC components (subcarrier at position 32) is not used. Pilot symbols are usually some known deterministic signals that are used for channel estimation and synchronization between transmitter and receiver. The guard intervals in OFDM systems are used to reduce the inter channel interference, and they are usually placed at the beginning and at the end of the spectrum.

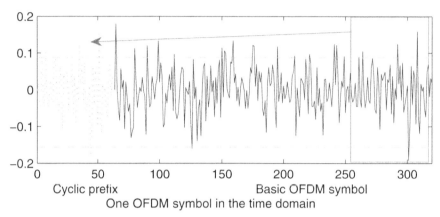

Figure 3 Time domain representation of an OFDM symbol, dotted line – cyclic prefix, solid line – basic OFDM symbol.

In order to obtain the OFDM symbol in the time domain, the inverse Fourier transform (IFFT block), is applied for each frequency bin:

$$s(t) = \frac{1}{\sqrt{N}} \sum_{k=0}^{N-1} A_k e^{(2\pi f_k t + \phi_k)}. \tag{2}$$

The output of the IFFT block is converted from serial to parallel stream, and the basic OFDM symbol of duration T_u is obtained (Figure 3). In order to avoid synchronization errors and to suppress inter symbol interference the cyclic prefix is added to the basic OFDM symbol. It is performed by copying last T_{cp} samples of the basic OFDM symbol to its beginning, as illustrated in Figure 3.

Finally, the D/A conversion is applied and the signal is amplified and transmitted.

OFDM demodulation requires the opposite procedure. After A/D conversion, the receiver discards the cyclic prefix and converts data from serial to parallel stream. The Fourier transform is then applied to recover the modulated symbols parameters. The output data stream is obtained after parallel to serial conversion and demodulation process.

3 Peak-to-Average Power Ratio Problem

A high peak-to-average power ratio is one of the problems in OFDM based transmission systems. It causes low energy efficiency of high-power amp-

Table 1 PAPR variations with respect to the number of subcarriers.

No. of carriers	64	128	256	512	1024	2048
Theoretical PAPR [dB]	18.06	21.07	24.08	27.09	30.1	33.11
PAPR for all carriers used [dB]	17.92	21	24.05	27.07	30.09	33.1
PAPR for 3/4 of carriers used [dB]	16.81	19.82	22.83	25.84	28.85	31.86
PAPR for 1/2 of carriers used [dB]	15.06	18.06	21.07	24.08	27.09	30.1
PAPR for 1/4 of carriers used [dB]	12.04	15.05	18.06	22.83	24.08	27.09

lifiers, D/A converters and other circuits used for transmission [1]. For the OFDM signal given by (2), the PAPR is defined as the ratio of maximal signal value and its average power:

$$\text{PAPR}(x(t)) = \frac{\max(|x(t)|^2)}{E\{|x(t)|^2\}}, \tag{3}$$

where $E\{\cdot\}$ denotes the expected value. Due to the multicarrier nature, random subcarrier's phases and random subcarrier's amplitudes (in the case of QAM modulation) the maximal value of an OFDM signal can become significant.

The PAPR is very sensitive regarding number of carriers used for data transmission. Namely, by increasing the number of subcarriers used for data transmission, the maximal signal value increases and causes high PAPR [1]. The PAPR values for the cases of 64, 128, 256, 512, 1024 and 2048 available subcarriers and for different numbers of used subcarriers are reported in Figure 4 and Table 1 (QPSK modulation is considered). In the case of QPSK modulation, each subcarrier has the constant amplitude $|A_k| = 1$, and the maximal theoretical PAPR value in digital domain can be calculated as [1, 4]:

$$\text{PAPR} = 10 \log 10(N). \tag{4}$$

Observe that PAPR increases by increasing the number of available and used subcarriers. Also, we can note that for the same number of available subcarriers PAPR decreases by reducing number of occupied subcarriers. However, it will also reduce the amount of data that can be transmitted within one OFDM symbol.

Beside the number of used subcarriers, the PAPR can be also influenced by the modulation scheme. The PAPR values for QPSK, 16QAM, 64QAM, and 256QAM modulation techniques are reported in Figure 5 and Table 2. One can observe that the PAPR is smallest in the case of QPSK, while it is largest for 256QAM.

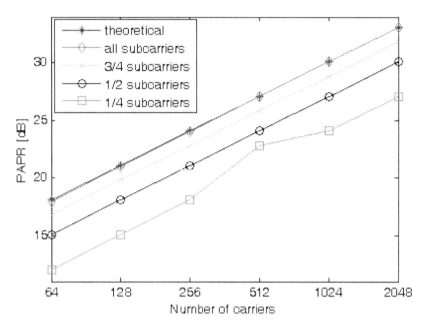

Figure 4 Influence of the number of subcarriers used for data transmission to the PAPR value.

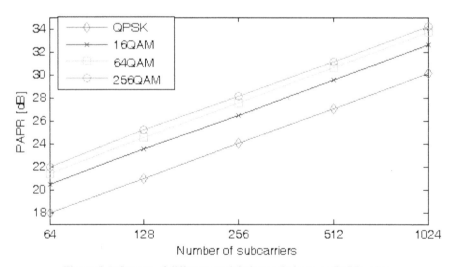

Figure 5 Influence of different modulation techniques to PAPR value.

Table 2 PAPR comparision for different modulation schemes.

No. of carriers	64	128	256	512	1024
PAPR for QPSK [dB]	17.92	21	24.05	27.07	30.09
PAPR for 16QAM [dB]	20.43	23.56	26.5	29.54	32.59
PAPR for 64QAM [dB]	21.38	24.56	27.57	30.66	33.7
PAPR for 256QAM [dB]	21.94	25.18	28.12	31.16	34.2

Table 3 Basic specifications of some OFDM based communication standards.

Application	Number of available subcarriers					Modulation
WLAN	64					BPSK, QPSK, 16QAM, or 64QAM
WiMAX	Fixed	Mobile Scalable	Mobile Scalable	Mobile Scalable	Mobile Scalable	BPSK, QPSK, 4,16,32,64, or 256QAM
	256	128	512	1024	2048	
DAB	Mode1	Mode2	Mode3	Mode4		DQPSK
	2048	512	256	1024		
DVB-T	2K Mode		8K Mode			QPSK, 16QAM or 64QAM
	2048		8192			
DVB-C	4096		8192		32768	64-QAM up to 4096-QAM

In order to analyze some real cases the total number of subcarriers and the type of modulation techniques for different OFDM based systems are reported in Table 3. According to the previous analysis we have that, for example, in WLAN systems (Table 4) with $N = 64$ subcarriers and QPSK modulation PAPR is 18 dB, while in WiMAX and DAB systems with $N = 256$ subcarriers and QPSK PAPR is 24 dB holds. Since the analog OFDM signals are fed to the amplifiers, the equivalent PAPRs in analog domain [4, 11], for real systems with $N = 64$ and $N = 256$ (with QPSK) are 12.1 and 18.1 dB, respectively. Similarly, for WLAN system with $N = 64$ and 64QAM the equivalent PAPR is 17.16 dB is obtained [1].

It is important to note that even the value of 12.1 dB (obtained for $N = 64$ and QPSK) is considered as high PAPR, because it implies that the peak value is more than one order of magnitude stronger than the average signal value. In real cases the PAPR is usually somewhat lower than the theoretical one, but it is still high and thus the OFDM systems require the so called PAPR reduction techniques. Some of these techniques are analyzed in the sequel.

4 Analysis of PAPR Reduction Techniques

In the previous section, the performances of OFDM systems have been analyzed with respect to the PAPR value. In order to obtain more precise

Table 4 Performances of different PAPR reduction techniques.

	System	IFFT size	Modulation		Threshold λ [dB]		CCDF [dB]	BER
					No clipping	Standard Clipping		
Clipping [6]	WiMaX	1024		BPSK	13.4	4.4	10^{-3}	10^{-1}
				4QAM	14.7	6.3		
				16QAM	14.9	7.8		
				64QAM	15.1	9.6		
				256QAM	15.4	10		
Selective mapping [7]	Wireless IEEE802.11a	64		BPSK	12			no distortion
				QPSK	11			
				DQPSK	9.8			
Selective mapping [8]	Unknown	128	QPSK (RSC turbo code with K=4)	2 bits code	9.8		10^{-3}	no distortion
				4 bits code	8.2			
				5 bits code	7.7			
				6 bits code	7			
Constellation manipulations [4]	WiMaX	256		No reduction	11.7		10^{-3}	no distortion
				QPSK	8.3			
				16QAM	9.8			
				64 QAM	10.6			
Modulation adaptation and clipping algorithm [6]	WiMaX	1024	BPSK+4QAM+16QAM +64QAM+256QAM		9 dB		10^{-3}	10^{-5}
Time and frequency swapping [5]	Unknown	256	4FSK	Clipp. level 80%	5.4		10^{-2}	
				Clipp. level 90%	5			
				Clipp. level 95%	4.6			
Sequential algorithm [5]	Unknown	256	4FSK		6.3		10^{-2}	no distortion
Partial transmit sequence with original cross-entropy method [10]	Unknown	128	QPSK	5 iterations	6.25		10^{-3}	no distortion
				17 iterations	6.04			

analysis, the performances of OFDM system can be evaluated with respect to the probability that PAPR is above some predefined threshold λ (in dB). As a measure of performances, the complementary cumulative distribution function (CCDF) is used:

$$\Pr\{PAPR > \lambda\} = 1 - (1 - e^{-\lambda})^N. \qquad (5)$$

Various techniques have been proposed in order to reduce PAPR in OFDM systems. Some of these techniques are: clipping and its modifications [5, 6]; partial transmit sequence [9, 10]; selective mapping [5, 7, 8]; constellations manipulations [4], etc. In the sequel we will consider some of these techniques and discuss their capabilities to reduce PAPR. The comparative results for different PAPR reduction techniques are summarized in Table 4. The characteristics of the applied PAPR reduction techniques are given in columns 2, 3, and 4. Column 5 contains the threshold values, while in the Column 6 the probabilities that PAPR exceeds specified threshold are reported.

Clipping is the simplest technique for PAPR reduction. It assumes that all amplitudes above predefined threshold λ are clipped to the threshold value. This value should be chosen to provide linear signal amplification and good power efficiency of high power amplifiers. For example, in WiMaX systems, the PAPR will be between 4.4 and 10 dB (depending on the modulation scheme) with the probability of 10^{-3}. However, the bit-error-rate (BER) is equal to 10^{-1} which is unacceptable in most of the applications. Thus, clipping based techniques may cause significant signal distortions and high BER.

An interesting modification of clipping technique is time and frequency swapping algorithm [5], where clipping is performed within a few iterative steps. In the first step, the random phases are assigned to each subcarrier and then transformed to time domain by using IFFT. The signal values are clipped in time domain and transformed back in the frequency domain. The procedure is repeated until the PAPR stops decreasing. It has been shown that, for $N = 256$ and 4FSK modulation, the probability that PAPR does not excide the range [4.6 dB, 5.4 dB] is 10^{-3} for clipping threshold between 80 and 95% of the maximal OFDM signal value. This system is characterized by high complexity and requires between 200 and 800 IFFT and FFT operations.

The algorithm based on modulation adaptation and clipping has been proposed in [6]. Based on predefined BER, the appropriate modulation is chosen for each sample. The clipping with high threshold value is applied to additionally reduce PAPR. The clipping is also used to control the switching between different modulation schemes. For this technique PAPR is 8 dB with probability 10^{-3}, while the BER is approximately 10^{-5}.

The sequential algorithm for PAPR reduction has been proposed in [5]. The different phases from the range $\{0, \pi\}$ are used to modify phases of used subcarriers. Modified signal is transformed in the time domain and PAPR is calculated. Then the phases are flipped and new PAPR is obtained. If the PAPR is not reduced, the original phases are kept. Probability that PAPR does not exceed value of 6.3 dB is approximately 10^{-2}. Although it provides worse performance compared to time and frequency swapping algorithm, the complexity of this system is much lower since it requires only 65 IFFT operations. Also, it does not introduce signal distortion, as it is the case with the time and frequency swapping or clipping techniques.

The partial transmission algorithm is another non-distortion technique [9, 10]. It divides the OFDM symbol into several shorter sequences that are separately optimized by using the cross-entropy method. The side information provided by the cross-entropy method should be sent to the receiver, which reduces the system capacity, i.e. the useful data rate.

Finally, the non-distortion solution based on selective mapping has been proposed in [5, 7, 8]. It uses additional bits to modify original sequence in a way to reduce PAPR. Namely, this algorithm iteratively adds different bits, while the lowest PAPR is obtained. The sequence that produces lowest PAPR is transmitted within OFDM symbol, and serves as side information at the receiver. By increasing number of bits used to modify original sequence, PAPR is reduced, but the channel utilization is decreased. For example, it has been shown in [8] that by using six bits to modify original sequence, PAPR can be reduced by 3 dB.

5 Conlusion

One of the main drawbacks of the OFDM based systems is high PAPR that causes high power consumption. Hence, these systems require some efficient PAPR reduction techniques. Generally, they can be classified into two categories: techniques that introduce signal distortion and non-distortion techniques. The techniques from the first group are usually much simpler and they can significantly reduce PAPR (e.g. PAPR is 4 dB in WiMAX systems) at the expense of lower signal quality. On the other hand, non-distortion techniques can provide limited PAPR reduction (in the best case the PARP can be reduced up to 6 dB). However, these techniques do not degrade the quality of original signal. Obviously, the compromise between PAPR reduction and signal quality should be made according to the specific application requirements. Finally, the PAPR reduction is still an open topic, since there is an increased demand for OFDM systems with improved energy efficiency, especially in mobile transmission systems.

References

[1] S. Kaiser. OFDM Code-Division Multiplexing in fading channels. *IEEE Transactions on Communications*, 50(8):1266–1273, August 2002.

[2] W. Shieh and I. Djordjevic. *OFDM for Optical Communications*. Academic Press, 2009.

[3] B. Debaillie, B. Bougard, G. Lenoir, G. Vandersteen, and F. Catthoor. Energy-scalable OFDM transmitter design and control. In *Proceedings of 43rd ACM/IEEE Design Automation Conference*, San Francisco, CA, pp. 536–541, 2006.

[4] C. Ciochina, F. Buda, and H. Sari. An analysis of OFDM peak power reduction techniques for WiMAX systems. In *Proceedings of IEEE International Conference on Communications ICC'06*, 10:4676–4681, June 2006.

[5] M. Wetz, W. Teich, and J. Lindner. PAPR reduction methods for noncoherent OFDM-MFSK. *Wireless Personal Communications*, 47:113–123, October 2008.

[6] I.I. Al-Kebsi, M. Ismail, K. Jumari, and T.A. Rahman. Mobile WiMaX performance improvement using a novel algorithm with a new form of adaptive modulation. *International Journal of Computer Science and Network Security*, 9(2):76–82, February 2009.

[7] V.B. Malode and B.P. Patil. Peak-to-average power ratio of OFDM system QPSK/DQPSK. In *Proceedings of the International Conference on Information Science and Applications ICISA 2010*, Chennai, India, February 2010.

[8] A.A. Abouda. PAPR reduction of OFDM signal using turbo coding and selective mapping. In *Proceedings of the 6th Nordic Signal Processing Symposium – NORSIG*, Espoo, Finland, June 2004.

[9] S.H. Müller and J.B. Huber. OFDM with reduced peak-to-average power ratio by optimum combination of partial transmit sequences. *Electron. Lett.*, 33(5):368–369, February 1997.

[10] J.-C. Chen. Partial transmit sequences for peak-to-average power ratio reduction of OFDM signals with the cross-entropy method. *IEEE Signal Processing Letters*, 16(6):545–548, June 2009.

[11] J. Tellado. *Multicarrier Modulation with Low Peak to Average Power Applications to xDSL and Broadband Wireless*. Kluwer Academic Publishers, Boston/Dordrecht/London, 2000.

Biographies

Irena Orović (S'06) was born in Montenegro in 1983. She received the B.Sc., M.Sc., and Ph.D. degrees in electrical engineering from the University of Montenegro, Podgorica, Montenegro, in 2005, 2006, and 2010, respectively. From 2005 to 2010, she was a Teaching Assistant with the University of Montenegro. Since 2010, she has been an Associate Professor with the Faculty of Electrical Engineering, University of Montenegro. Her research interests include multimedia systems, digital watermarking, and time-frequency analysis.

Nikola Žarić was born in Montenegro in 1982. He received his B.Sc., M.Sc. and Ph.D. degrees in electrical engineering from the University of Montenegro, Montenegro, in 2005, 2006, and 2010, respectively. Since 2005, he has been employed as a Teaching Assistant at the Faculty of Electrical Engineering, University of Montenegro. In October 2010 he was promoted to Associate Professor at the Faculty of Electrical Engineering, University of Montenegro. His research interests are in digital watermarking and time-frequency analysis and related hardware realizations.

Srdjan Stanković was born in Montenegro in 1964. He received his B.S. (Hons.) degree in electrical engineering from the University of Montenegro, in 1988, his M.S. degree in electrical engineering from the University of Zagreb, Croatia, in 1991, and his Ph.D. degree in electrical engineering from the University of Montenegro in 1993. He is a Full Professor at the Faculty of Electrical Engineering, University of Montenegro. Since 2007, he has been the Dean of the Faculty of Electrical Engineering, University of Montenegro. His interests are in signal processing, multimedia systems, and digital electronics. He was the President of the Board of Directors in Montenegrin Broadcasting Company (2005–2006). In 1998 he spent a period of time with the Department of Informatics at the Aristotle University in Thessaloniki, supported by Greek IKY foundation. From 1999 to 2000, he was on leave at the Darmstadt University of Technology, with the Signal Theory Group, supported by the Alexander von Humboldt Foundation. In 2002, he spent three months at the Department of Computer Science, the University of Applied Sciences Bonn-Rhein-Sieg, as an Alexander von Humboldt Fellow. From 2004 to 2006, he stayed several times with the E^3I^2 Lab, ENSIETA, Brest. From 2007 to 2009 he visited (one month research stay) the Centre for Digital Signal Processing Research at King's College London, the Laboratory of Mathematical Methods of Image Processing, at Moscow State University Lomonosov, CAC at Villanova University PA, and the GIPSA Laboratory at INPG Grenoble. He has published several textbooks on electronics devices (in Montenegrin) and coauthored a monograph on time-frequency signal analysis (in English). He has published more than 100 papers in the areas of signal and image processing.

He is the Leading Guest Editor of the *EURASIP Journal on Advances in Signal Processing* special issue on "Time-frequency analysis and its applications to multimedia signals", as well as Guest Editor of the *Signal Processing* special issue on "Fourier related transforms".

From 2005 to 2009 Dr. Stanković served as an Associate Editor of the *IEEE Transactions on Image Processing*.

Igor Radusinovic, born in Montenegro in 1972, received his B.Sc. degree in electrical engineering from the University of Montenegro, Montenegro, in 1994. He received his M.Sc. and Ph.D. degrees in electrical engineering from the University of Belgrade, Serbia in 1997, and 2003, respectively. From 1994 to 2003, he was a Teaching Assistant with the University of Montenegro. From 2003 to 2008, he was an Assistant Professor with the

University of Montenegro. Since 2008, he has been an Associate Professor with the Faculty of Electrical Engineering, University of Montenegro. He has served as a reviewer for leading scientific journals in the different areas of telecommunications, as well as a member of Programme Committees of several conferences. His research interests are mainly in telecommunications network protocols and systems design. His current research topics are packet switch architectures, quality of service in wired/wireless networks, green communications and congestion control. In these areas he has published more than 100 referred publications in peer-review international journals and international proceedings.

Zoran Veljović was born in Serbia in 1968. He received his B.Sc. degree in electrical engineering from the University of Montenegro in 1992, his M.Sc. degree in electrical engineering from the University of Belgrade, Serbia, in 1997, and his Ph.D. degree in electrical engineering from the University of Montenegro in 2005. From 1992 to 2006, he was a Teaching Assistant with the University of Montenegro. Since 2006, he has been an Assistant Professor with the Faculty of Electrical Engineering, University of Montenegro. Since 2007 he has been Vice Dean for Academic Affairs. His research interests are mainly in digital communication systems, digital modulations, and mobile, satellite optical and maritime communications.

Author Index, Volume 1 (2011)

Aghvami, A.H., 355
Alexandru, A., 111
Atanasovski, V., 241
Athanasiou, G., 383
Banciu, D., 111
Bazzani, A., 67
Boscovic, D., 33
Calvanese Strinati, E., 267
Chiani, M., 431
Çetin, B.K., 189
Cimmino, A., 255
Condeixa, T., 329
Coutinho, N., 329
Dado, M., 55
De Domenico, A., 267
del Camino Noguera, M., 355
Demestichas, P., 1, 383
Donadio, P., 255
Gavrilovska, L., 241
Giorgetti, A., 431
Giorgini, B., 67
Gupta, P.K., 145
Havelka, J., 179
Herault, L., 267
Holland, O., 355
Hooli, B., 89
Janota, A., 55
Karvounas, D., 383
Kljaić, Z., 413

Kokkinaki, A., 165
Koutitas, G., 1
Kritikou, Y., 383
Larsen, P.G., 303
Lindgren, P., 229
Logothetis, M., 383
Louca, S., 165
Lux, D., 303
Mandzuka, S., 413
Minardi, S., 431
Misra, P., 89
Murakami, M., 89
Namboodiri, V., 447
Needham, M., 33
Neto, A., 329
Orović, I., 477
Pais, N., 189
Paolini, E., 431
Pavić, I., 179
Pierson, J.-M., 129
Prasad, A.R., 89
Prasad, N.R., 189
Prasad, R., 189, 209, 255
Pratas, N., 189
Radusinović, I., 477
Rakovic, V., 241
Rambaldi, S., 67
Rovsing, P.E., 303
Saha, S., 89

Sargento, S., 329
Šimić, Z., 179
Šimunic, D., 209
Singh, G., 145
Skjødeberg Toftegaard, T., 303
Škorput, P., 413
Somovat, P., 447
Spalek, J., 55
Stanković, S., 477

Taran, Y., 229
Tsagkaris, K., 383
Vakil, F., 33
Velez, F.J., 189, 355
Veljović, Z., 477
Yang, J., 33
Žarić, N., 477
Zrno, D., 209

Keyword Index, Volume 1 (2011)

ad-hoc networks, 209
automatic meter reading, 431
automation, 179
broadband communication, 355
business model, 229
Cell Broadcasting, 413
cell zooming, 355
climate change, 111
cloud, 129
cloud computing, 255
clusters, 129
cognitive management, 383
cognitive networks, 209
computing, 447
Content Delivery Network (CDN), 33
context-awareness, 329
cooperative systems, 179
data center carbon footprint combination, 1
data center design, 1
Data Center Performance Efficiency (DCPE), 33
distributed control, 179
EARTH, 267
ecological impact 129
economics, 355
E-governance, 67
eLearning, 111

electricity, 447
energy education, 111
energy efficiency, 229, 267
energy efficiency of data center, 1
energy efficient metrics, 1
energy management, 179
energy, 447
energy-aware, 383
energy saving, 111, 303, 431
environment, 55, 447
femtocells, 267
future networks, 383
GHG, 89
GISFI, 89
green, 89
green business models, 229
green communications, 267, 355
green computing, 329
green footprint, 383
green society, 229
green supply chain management, 165
greenhouse gas (GHG), 145
heterogeneity, 329
heterogeneous network, 431
heterogeneous wireless networks, 229
home automation, 303
hybrid energy storage system, 189
ICT, 89

IEEE 802.21, 229
Incident Management System, 413
information and communication
　technology, 55, 179
innovation, 229
intelligent power profile (IPP), 145
intelligent transport system, 55
intelligent transportation systems,
　413
interference, 209, 267
interoperability, 303
location based broadcasting, 413
low energy complex systems, 67
multicast, 329
network management, 255
networking, 447
next generation networks, 255
OFDM, 477
opportunistic networks, 383
overlay, 329
peak-to-average power ratio, 477
planning, 355
portable devices 447
power consumption, 145
power system economics, 179
powerline communications, 431
protocols, 303
quality of service, 329

radio resource management, 267
rechargeable battery, 189
re-lays, 355
remote control, 431
renewable energy sources, 111
resource management, 229
reverse logistics, 165
routing protocol, 189
Service Oriented Architecture
　(SOA), 255
Service Oriented Infrastructure
　(SOI), 255
SLAM, 209
smart routing, 209
supercapacitor, 189
task allocation, 129
throughput, 209
traffic engineering, 383
transmission systems, 477
urban mobility, 67
Video on Demand (VoD), 33
virtualization, 255
volatile organic compounds (VOCs),
　145
WiMAX, 355
wireless, 303
wireless networks, 209
wireless sensor networks, 189

Online Manuscript Submission

The link for submission is: www.riverpublishers.com/journal

Authors and reviewers can easily set up an account and log in to submit or review papers.

Submission formats for manuscripts: LaTeX, Word, WordPerfect, RTF, TXT.
Submission formats for figures: EPS, TIFF, GIF, JPEG, PPT and Postscript.

LaTeX

For submission in LaTeX, River Publishers has developed a River stylefile, which can be downloaded from http://riverpublishers.com/river_publishers/authors.php

Guidelines for Manuscripts

Please use the Authors' Guidelines for the preparation of manuscripts, which can be downloaded from http://riverpublishers.com/river_publishers/authors.php

In case of difficulties while submitting or other inquiries, please get in touch with us by clicking CONTACT on the journal's site or sending an e-mail to: info@riverpublishers.com

www.ingramcontent.com/pod-product-compliance
Lightning Source LLC
LaVergne TN
LVHW012331060326
832902LV00011B/1824